the DOCTOR'S DIET

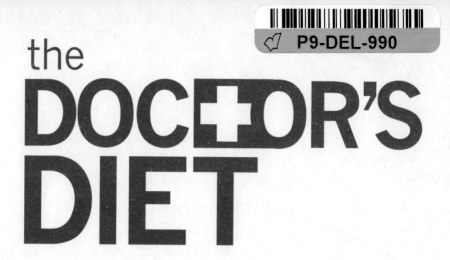

Dr. Travis Stork's **STAT** Program to Help You
Lose Weight & Restore Health

By **TRAVIS STORK, MD**

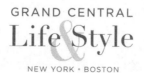

GRAND CENTRAL
Life & Style
NEW YORK · BOSTON

Grand Central Life & Style
Hachette Book Group
1290 Avenue of the Americas
New York, NY 10104
www.GrandCentralLifeandStyle.com

Printed in the United States of America

RRD-C

First Grand Central Life & Style trade paperback edition: December 2015

10 9 8 7 6 5 4 3 2 1

Grand Central Life & Style is an imprint of Grand Central Publishing.
The Grand Central Life & Style name and logo is a trademark of Hachette Book Group, Inc.

The Hachette Speakers Bureau provides a wide range of authors for speaking events.
To find out more, go to www.hachettespeakersbureau.com or call (866) 376-6591.

The publisher is not responsible for websites (or their content)
that are not owned by the publisher.

Layout by Stuart Smith

LCCN 2015950583

ISBN 978-1-4555-3821-8 (pbk.)

Dedicated to all of those in search of health and happiness.

ACKNOWLEDGMENTS

I want to personally thank Alice Lesch Kelly for her enthusiasm and dedication to this project, and Lisa Clark for her guidance every step of the way. To Jon Ford, Ashlee Gagui, Hagop Kalaidjian, Maggie Greenwood-Robinson, and everyone else who played a role in putting this book together: I thank you!

CONTENTS

INTRODUCTION
THE WEIGHT GAIN EMERGENCY

Lights flash. Sirens blare. An emergency services vehicle rushes through the streets in a life-or-death race against time. Inside the ambulance, emergency medical technicians work frantically to stabilize their patient. Screeching to a halt, the EMTs throw open the ambulance doors, grab the gurney on which their patient lies, and charge into the emergency room. There, highly trained ER doctors and nurses take over, springing into action in a tenacious fight for the patient's life. When luck is on their side, the patient pulls through. When it's not, an ER doctor is left with the heartbreaking task of having to deliver the tragic news of the patient's death to their family.

Too many times, I have been the ER doc giving this awful news. No matter how many times it happens, it never gets any easier to tell someone that the person who means more to them than anyone else in the world—their mom, their dad, their sister, their brother, their child—has passed away. I feel as if I lose a little piece of my heart every time I have to do it.

What makes it toughest is knowing that so many untimely deaths could have been prevented.

Death is inevitable, of course. No matter how hard we try, we can't avoid it. But death isn't always a tragedy. When someone who's lived a long, happy life dies peacefully at home, surrounded by family and friends, that's terribly sad, of course. But it's not a tragedy. When someone's life ends years or even decades before it should? When someone's quality of life is compromised at an early age? That's a tragedy. And that's the kind of death and disability that ER docs see every single day.

When you think about all of these unnecessary ER deaths, you may shudder as you imagine their causes—horrible trauma, grisly accidents, car crashes, even gun violence.

But when it comes to the kinds of problems we see most often in the ER, the reality is actually quite different than what most people imagine.

THE BIGGEST EMERGENCY IN ERs ACROSS THE UNITED STATES IS THE FOOD WE WILLINGLY, KNOWINGLY, HAPPILY CHOOSE TO EAT.

NOT AN ACCIDENT

The majority of patients in ERs are not there because of trauma or accidents. They are there because of their diets. That's right: the biggest emergency in ERs across the United States is the food we willingly, knowingly, happily choose to eat.

Our food choices are so dangerously unhealthy that eating-related diseases send *twice as many people* to hospital ERs than injuries and accidents.

Unhealthy eating contributes to as many as 580,000 deaths in the United States every year. That's more than smoking, drug abuse, gun violence, and traffic accidents *combined*. If you eat the typical American diet, it very well may kill you.

I don't want that to happen to you! As an ER doctor and as a fellow human being who loves life with an infinite passion, I want to protect you from that fate. I don't want YOU to be the person on the gurney being rushed to the hospital with flashing lights and blaring sirens. I don't want YOU to be the patient lying in the ER with a medical team fighting desperately to save your life. I don't want YOU to be the corpse wheeled to the morgue while an ER doctor gives your shocked family the tragic news that you are gone forever because your life could not be saved.

I'm not telling you this to scare you. Quite the opposite—I'm leveling with you because I care about you. I want to empower you. I want to energize you and give you hope! As bad as this black cloud of health facts sounds, it actually has a really amazing silver lining. It doesn't have to happen to you! You don't have to be the dying ER patient with a distraught family. You can turn your diet around, and in doing so, you can revive your health and change your life.

That's right. No matter how bad your diet is, no matter how much excess weight you're carrying around, no matter how many food-related mistakes you've made in the past, you can start fresh *now*. You can embark on a new way of living *today* that will immediately begin to chip away at your risk of dying from your diet.

How? By following The Doctor's Diet.

It's that simple. Changes that you can start to make *right this minute* can turn your diet from a flashing-lights emergency to a health-boosting, life-saving gift that you give yourself and your family. You really can turn your life around—and The Doctor's Diet can show you how.

> ✚ OUR FOOD CHOICES ARE SO DANGEROUSLY UNHEALTHY THAT EATING-RELATED DISEASES SEND TWICE AS MANY PEOPLE TO HOSPITAL ERs THAN INJURIES AND ACCIDENTS.

DELICIOUS CHANGES

Change can be difficult—believe me, I understand that. It's hard to let go of a lifetime of poor eating habits and grab on to a healthy new diet. But I promise you, with The Doctor's Diet, I'm making it as easy for you as possible. I've created a program that will guide you, step by step, in the simplest way possible, to develop a healthier dietary outlook that will help you lose weight, restore your health, reduce disease risk, and pave the way for you to live a longer, happier life.

The Doctor's Diet is way more than just an eating plan—it's a blueprint for a longer, healthier, happier life. It's everything you need to know to keep yourself OUT of the ER.

But don't worry: as we travel together down the path to better health, I'm not going to ask you to eat bland, boring "diet" food. Listen, I'm a man who loves food. I absolutely cannot make a meal out of a giant bowl of raw broccoli—to tell you the truth, eating straight-up veggies like that is about as appealing to me as sitting down to a plate of swamp grass and acorns. I grew up in the Midwest, raised on bacon and eggs for breakfast, big sandwiches for lunch, and meat and potatoes for dinner. Vegetables were an afterthought, and more often than not they came from a can. My idea of a snack was a football-sized burrito or as many brownies as I could fit in my hands—and these mitts are pretty big, so that's a lot of brownies.

As I got older and started tasting food from other parts of the United States and the world, I fell in love with exciting new flavors and delicious new foods. And as I spent year after grueling year training to become a physician, I learned about the strength of the link between food and wellness. So believe me, I love good health. But I also love to eat, and I am not about to tell you (or myself) that a healthy diet has to be boring or tasteless.

FOODS YOU CAN LIVE WITH

Switching from low-nutrient foods (white bread, processed meats, chips, cookies, and so on) to the super-nutritious foods included in The Doctor's Diet does take some getting used to—I understand that. When you're accustomed to having a greasy burger with fries for lunch, for example, it may seem strange to sit down to a meal made up of vegetables, healthy protein, and whole grains.

Let me give you some reassurance on this. Yeah, the food in The Doctor's Diet may not be what you're used to. But believe me when I tell you you're going to love it.

I'll tell you a story. When I first started hosting *The Doctors*, the caterers who provided lunch for our first photo shoot brought in the usual fast-food fare. I took one look at it and realized we needed to make a change—here I was hosting a medical show about health, and the food we were eating was far from healthy. I had to speak up.

Since that time, the caterers have started serving the most delicious, healthiest food you can imagine. And I'm not the only one who loves it—the crew goes crazy over it, too. I always laugh to myself when I see these big guys—the ones who help build the sets and such—devouring a dish with salmon or chicken, quinoa, and veggies served with a spicy curry sauce. This is Doctor's Diet food, but they're not eating it because they're watching their weight—they're eating it because it tastes incredible.

I think you're going to love it as much as they do—and as much as I do.

I live The Doctor's Diet, and I eat the food I'm encouraging you to eat. I'm not about to tell you to put something on your plate that I wouldn't have on mine!

YOU CAN TURN YOUR DIET AROUND, AND IN DOING SO, YOU CAN REVIVE YOUR HEALTH AND CHANGE YOUR LIFE.

My program is designed to help you eat the foods you love, but to eat them in a healthy way that will add vibrancy to your life and help keep you out of the ER. Those big burritos I mentioned? I've put together my own burrito recipe that is about ten times healthier than those fast-food bombs I used to eat, and you know what? They're also about ten times tastier, too. Those handfuls of brownies I used to scarf down? Well, I still have a brownie now and then—total deprivation doesn't work for me, and research shows it doesn't work for most other people, either.

But I've learned that adding a dollop of mindfulness to an occasional treat makes it way more enjoyable and satisfying than a handful gobbled up thoughtlessly. That's why mindfulness—developing an awareness of what you're eating so you can fully enjoy its flavor—is one of the many new mindsets you'll learn in my program that will help you taste and savor healthy food in a whole new way.

THE NUMBER OF PEOPLE WITH TYPE 2 DIABETES IS EXPECTED TO RISE SHARPLY DURING THE COMING DECADES. UNLESS WE MAKE SOME BIG CHANGES TO OUR DIETS AND ACTIVITY LEVELS, BY 2050, AS MANY AS ONE-THIRD OF ADULTS WILL HAVE TYPE 2 DIABETES (UP FROM 8.3 PERCENT TODAY).

Just as flavor is a big part of The Doctor's Diet, so is medical integrity. My most important professional role in life is being a physician. When I swore the Hippocratic oath—as every doctor does—I promised to practice medicine honestly and without harm to patients. I take that oath very seriously. You can be sure that all of my advice and recommendations are based on my full commitment to your health.

My program is not a gimmicky fad diet based on the latest pseudo-science. It is an evidence-based plan that is grounded in nutritional science. Every recommendation and guideline is backed by solid research that you can trust, and by my sacred oath as a physician. That's my promise to you.

Come along with me on this journey to optimal health and I'll do everything in my power to make sure you live a long, vibrant life. Decide now to commit to an eating plan that could very well save your life. Don't wait until you're lying in the ER, praying for a second chance. Do it now, before it's too late!

GETTING STARTED
ABOUT THIS BOOK

I've been thinking about writing a book of dietary advice for some time. But I didn't want it to be like all the other diet books out there—I truly want my plan to be the ultimate diet plan, one that rises head and shoulders above all the others not only because of its medical integrity, but because of its simplicity and its effectiveness. As a physician, I don't believe in gimmicky, get-slim-quick schemes. I believe in an eating plan that leads not only to weight loss, but to an exciting new level of health and vitality that you simply can't get by following crazy crash diets. The Doctor's Diet is the real deal.

This book tells you everything you need to do, step by step, meal by meal, day by day, to lose excess weight and build robust health. It is absolutely loaded with tips that you can use in your daily life—tips that require minimal effort but provide huge health benefits with one goal in mind: to motivate you to live your best, happiest, and healthiest life.

Following The Doctor's Diet is the closest thing to having me by your side throughout the day, guiding your choices, helping you on your journey to better health, a longer life, and yes—to looking better in your swimsuit.

It won't take nearly as much effort as you might think, but it will take one very important thing: commitment. So I'm asking you today, at this very moment in time, to commit to making the potentially life-saving changes in your diet and activity levels that I recommend in this book. If you commit, then I promise you the pages that follow will give you the simple tools you need to make better, life-changing choices.

One of the things I'm constantly trying to do as a physician is to convince people that the food they put in their mouths today truly will affect how well and how long they live. These days, we have the latest medical technology and access to all kinds of cutting-edge medications that are extending our lives. But too many people who live longer suffer for years at the ends of their lives because of disease-related disability. We may be living for more years, but how many of those years are filled with vibrancy?

By following The Doctor's Diet, you will be taking giant steps toward living a life that is not only longer, but better—a life filled with friends, family, fun, and laughter rather than debilitating disease, hospitals, nursing homes, and worry.

The Doctor's Diet is based on the lessons that have guided me throughout my own journey to optimal health. It is exactly what I recommend to any patient, family member, or friend looking for a way to feel better, drop extra weight, and reduce disease risk. The lessons in this book have helped me and so many others, and I look forward to them helping you as well!

> I'M ASKING YOU TODAY, AT THIS VERY MOMENT IN TIME, TO COMMIT TO HAVING A BETTER, HEALTHIER LIFE. IF YOU COMMIT, THEN I PROMISE YOU THE PAGES THAT FOLLOW WILL GIVE YOU THE SIMPLE TOOLS YOU NEED TO MAKE BETTER, LIFE-CHANGING CHOICES. AND I'LL BE WITH YOU EVERY STEP OF THE WAY WITH THE ADVICE, INFORMATION, AND ENCOURAGEMENT YOU NEED TO SUCCEED.

THE DOCTOR'S PLAN FOR HEALTH AND LIFE

I'm sure you're raring to get started on The Doctor's Diet. But before we get down to the nitty-gritty, let's talk about what you can expect.

We'll start with the actual eating plan. In a nutshell, The Doctor's Diet is a science-based diet that:

+ Is low in sugar, simple carbohydrates, unhealthy fats, and sodium.

+ Includes moderate amounts of lean protein, healthy fats, and whole grains.

+ Contains generous amounts of fiber-rich vegetables, legumes, and fruits.

+ Is a "flexitarian" approach that allows everyone—whether you love meat or prefer to eat vegetarian, whether you have no time to cook or consider yourself a seasoned gourmet chef, whether you eat gluten-free or love Mediterranean cooking—to enjoy the food you love while losing weight and restoring robust health.

+ Abandons the all-or-nothing thinking that most diets embrace. I won't tell you that you "always" have to do this or "never" can do that. I'll give you the facts, offer my advice, and let you decide what's best for you. I know medicine, but you know your own body better than anyone else.

+ Answers your dietary questions based on current science—even if the answer to a question is "we don't know for sure." We know so much about nutrition science these days, but in a few areas, the research isn't completely clear on how certain foods affect our bodies. If the jury is still out on something, I'll be straight with you, and you can make your own choices based on what is and isn't known.

+ Recognizes that you have a limited amount of time in your life to spend on food preparation. My meal suggestions and recipes are simple and quick to prepare, calling for ingredients that you probably either have on hand or can easily pick up at your local grocery store.

+ Focuses on flavor, because life is too short to eat tasteless food!

+ Includes zesty herbs and spices such as ginger, chili powder, and hot sauces that have been shown in research to help incinerate body fat and ignite metabolism.

+ Relies on whole, natural foods prepared in ways that are filling, satisfying, and delicious.

+ Definitely does not rely on processed "diet" foods that are stripped of their natural ingredients and reconfigured with fake substitutions. I'd rather have you eat a small amount of real cheese, for example, than a big chunk of that horrible, chemical-filled, fat-free "cheese food" that so many diets call for.

+ Resets your taste buds by weaning you off junky, sugary, artificial foods and reintroducing you to the delicious, natural flavors in whole, unadulterated foods.

+ Advises you on smart snacking, choosing filling foods, and finding other ways to cut back on calories without feeling hungry all the time.

+ Gives you loads and loads of choices—because I don't like being told exactly what to eat every day, and I doubt you do, either.

+ Trades deprivation for moderation—because sometimes it's nice to have a treat.

SPOTLIGHT ON BELLY FAT

Burning away excess belly fat is a major goal of The Doctor's Diet. That's not because it's unattractive—although let's face it, we all care about how we look. As a doctor, I care about belly fat because having excess fat around your middle is dangerous for your overall health.

Also known as "visceral fat," belly fat is not just a benign bulge around your waist. In fact, it's very metabolically active—which means it contributes to how your body functions every day. Belly fat can harm you by releasing fatty acids into your blood, pumping out inflammatory agents, and producing hormones that wreak havoc on your body.

What's more, belly fat puts demands on your heart because it requires a constant infusion of oxygenated blood pumped by your heart. The more fat you have stored (in your belly and throughout your body), the harder your heart has to pump. Over time, this can dangerously strain your heart. Belly fat also threatens your heart by raising LDL cholesterol, triglycerides, blood sugar, and blood pressure.

You CAN banish your belly fat! The Doctor's Diet gives you all the tools you need to burn it off and keep it off.

The good news is overweight and obese people often find that once they start to shed pounds, the fat around their belly is some of the first to disappear. Science tells us that specific foods such as yogurt, as well as calcium-rich foods, omega-3 fats in fish, and whole grains truly do trim your belly fat, thanks to their effect on hormones and metabolism. As soon as you start following The Doctor's Diet, the fat around your middle will begin burning away.

START FEELING BETTER IMMEDIATELY

Following The Doctor's Diet can do incredible things for your long-term health, like lowering your risk of developing the kinds of chronic diseases that send people to the emergency room. As a doctor, that makes me ecstatic. But The Doctor's Diet isn't just about long-term benefits. Once you begin eating The Doctor's Diet way, you'll start noticing changes in how you feel *immediately*.

I know that sounds like a promise that can't be kept. You may be thinking, "Dr. Travis, how is it possible to start feeling better *right away?*"

Here's how: As soon as you commit to a healthier way of living, and as soon as you eat your first Doctor's Diet meal, you're going to begin feeling great about yourself.

Let me give you an example of this. Recently I chatted with someone who ate her first STAT Plan breakfast: a cup of blueberries, a scrambled egg, and half a cup of oatmeal sprinkled with chopped walnuts. (More on the STAT Plan soon.) It was the first time in years she'd eaten such a nutritious breakfast—usually her go-to was a bacon, egg, and cheese breakfast biscuit and a sweetened coffee drink from her local drive-thru donut shop.

Even before she finished her berries, she started feeling better about herself—not because her weight had suddenly dropped or her heart dis-ease risk disappeared, but because she realized that she had taken such a big first step on the road to good health.

Listen, one cup of berries and a bowl of oatmeal with nuts won't reverse the effects of years of breakfast biscuits. But it can be the meal that changes everything—it can be the breakfast that you look back on as the first meal of your new, healthier life.

Just knowing that you're making changes that will lead to weight loss and better health can be incredibly empowering! It can make you *feel* healthier even before you actually *are* healthier, and that's great, because the positive feeling you get in response to starting The Doctor's Diet can fuel you. It can encourage you to make the right choices at other meals, it can give you the energy to go for your daily walk, and it can give you blasts of motivation that will keep you jazzed until the pounds really do start dropping off.

SO MUCH MORE THAN WEIGHT LOSS

Although I know your number one goal might be to lose weight, The Doctor's Diet is much more than a weight-loss plan. This plan is not just about cutting calories—heck, you can lose weight eating cookies all day, so long as you limit your calories. To really, truly boost your health—and stay out of the ER—you have to go beyond weight loss and eat foods that support every cell of your body in a healthful, life-giving way. By taking a whole-health approach, you can do way more than just lose weight and trim your waist. Sure, you want to look great. But won't it be nice to know that you'll be boosting your health while whittling away your waist?

Losing weight and eating a healthy, life-supporting diet are two of the best things you can do for your health. Don't be discouraged if you've been unsuccessful in past efforts to shed excess pounds and change your diet. The Doctor's Diet is a different kind of eating plan, one that you can stick with for the rest of your life. It's not just a diet but a new way of life and a new way of eating. The Doctor's Diet is unique because it includes many of the foods you already eat, so there's no need to learn an entirely new way of cooking and preparing meals. The recipes and meal plans don't call for crazy ingredients and unusual foods that cost a bundle online or at specialty grocery stores. Rather, familiar foods are combined in a new way, using specially designed Meal Plan Equations that optimize fat burn and weight loss. Yeah, I'll ask you to try some new foods—super-nutritious foods that can boost your health and whittle away weight—but they're all foods that you can buy at your supermarket, prepare easily, and enjoy eating for the rest of your (long) life.

Not only that, but The Doctor's Diet also gives you a personal physician: me. As you set out on your journey to better health and longer life, I'll be with you every step of the way, giving you the information, advice, encouragement, and motivation you need to succeed.

With this book in your hands, everything you need is at your fingertips.

USING THE DOCTOR'S DIET MEAL PLAN EQUATIONS

The Doctor's Diet meals are built around unique daily Meal Plan Equations that rev up your metabolism, accelerate fat burn, and lead to high-octane weight loss. Each day, your meals and snacks are planned according to easy-to-remember Meal Plan Equations. This fantastic meal-planning tool shows you how to combine protein, certain types of carbohydrates, healthy fats, fruits, and various vegetables into each meal and snack—simply, and without counting calories.

When you plan your meals according to my Meal Plan Equations, you get the right balance of nutrients—protein, carbohydrates, healthy fats, vitamins, minerals, antioxidants, and everything else you need for great health, maximum fat burn, and speedy weight loss. Plus, you get delicious, satisfying meals that give you loads of energy.

DETERMINING YOUR GOAL WEIGHT

The best way to figure out your healthiest goal weight is to talk with your doctor. But in general, the research suggests that it's best to aim for a body-mass index (BMI) in the low to mid 20s.

BMI is a number calculated using a person's height and weight. Doctors use BMI as a guide to whether people are underweight, normal weight, overweight, or obese. BMI is not a 100 percent accurate way of determining goal weights, because it doesn't take into account the size of your frame or the amount of muscle you have. Muscle is denser than fat, so a very muscular person who has a perfectly healthy weight can have a BMI in the overweight range. But in general, doctors use BMI as a starting point for a discussion about goal weight.

Use the chart below to determine your BMI. Once you have it, check the BMI guide to see where your weight falls.

		19	20	21	22	23	24	25	26	27	28	29	30
						WEIGHT (LBS.)							
HEIGHT	4'10"	91	96	100	105	110	115	119	124	129	134	138	143
	4'11"	94	99	104	109	114	119	124	128	133	138	143	148
	5'	97	102	197	112	118	123	128	133	138	143	148	153
	5'1"	100	106	111	116	122	127	132	137	143	148	153	158
	5'2"	104	109	115	120	126	131	136	142	147	153	158	164
	5'3"	107	113	118	124	130	135	141	146	152	158	163	169
	5'4"	110	116	122	128	134	140	145	151	157	163	169	174
	5'5"	114	120	126	132	138	144	150	156	162	168	174	180
	5'6"	118	124	130	136	142	148	155	161	167	173	179	186
	5'7"	121	127	134	140	146	153	159	166	172	178	185	191
	5'8"	125	131	138	144	151	158	164	171	177	184	190	197
	5'9"	128	135	142	149	155	162	169	176	182	189	196	203
	5'10"	132	139	146	153	160	167	174	181	188	195	202	209
	5'11"	136	143	150	157	165	172	179	186	193	200	208	215
	6'	140	147	154	162	169	177	184	191	199	206	213	221
	6'1"	144	151	159	166	174	182	189	197	204	212	219	227
	6'2"	148	155	163	171	179	186	194	202	210	218	225	233
	6'3"	152	160	168	176	184	192	200	208	216	224	232	240
	6'4"	156	164	172	180	189	197	205	213	221	230	238	246

BMI	WEIGHT CATEGORY
Less than 18.5	Underweight
18.5 to 24.9	Normal Weight
25 to 29.9	Overweight
30 and over	Obese

THE DOCTOR'S DIET GAME PLAN

I've designed this book to give you everything you need to make life-saving changes that will keep you out of the ER and fully, vibrantly engaged in your healthy new life. To make things easy, I've structured The Doctor's Diet in this way:

PART ONE: GETTING STARTED WITH THE DOCTOR'S DIET 14-DAY STAT PLAN

You'll jump right into the Doctor's Diet with the STAT Plan. When someone is wheeled into the ER on the edge of death, the medical team leaps into action right away. The medical phrase for this is "STAT," from the Latin word *statim*, which means *immediately*. You've probably seen doctors on television use this word while barking orders to nurses—for example, "inject 1 mg of epinephrine STAT!"

In a medical emergency we rush to administer life-saving medications. When weight is an emergency, the same immediate action is called for. We want to start making health-boosting changes STAT. That's why I call the first phase of my eating plan the STAT Plan.

We're starting with the STAT Plan right away. No need to wait—just flip to page 30, and you can start following it at your *very next meal*. Seriously! Excess weight is a true emergency, and you can start your "treatment" right away.

Sure, I do want to explain everything about it to you eventually—for example, I want you to understand why I'm suggesting berries at breakfast or lentils at lunch—but I don't want you to have to spend hours or days reading about your new eating plan before you dive in. And I want you to get a thumbs-up from your own health-care provider before you make any major changes to your diet, especially if you have heart disease, diabetes, or any other health problems. But otherwise, there's no reason not to get started right away—STAT!

Think of it this way: When someone is wheeled into the emergency room having a heart attack, the medical team doesn't sit down with them and chat for a few hours about the structure of the heart and the finer points of myocardial infarction. We jump into action, administering cardiopulmonary resuscitation, infusing medications, sometimes rushing them off to the operating room for surgery. And we do it all with lightning speed—STAT.

The same goes for weight-loss emergencies. Being overweight or obese is a major health emergency that requires your immediate action. Not an emergency administration of drugs, medical procedures, or surgery, but an immediate change in your diet. If your weight is an emergency, you can start giving it emergency treatment right now by diving in to The Doctor's Diet STAT Plan right away.

BEING OVERWEIGHT OR OBESE IS A MAJOR HEALTH EMERGENCY THAT REQUIRES YOUR IMMEDIATE ACTION. NOT AN EMERGENCY ADMINISTRATION OF DRUGS, MEDICAL PROCEDURES, OR SURGERY, BUT AN IMMEDIATE CHANGE IN YOUR DIET.

WHAT YOU CAN EXPECT FROM THE DOCTOR'S DIET STAT PLAN

Using my high-intensity 14-day STAT Plan, you'll see *immediate* results. Within two weeks, you'll:

✚ Lose weight rapidly (up to 10 pounds in 14 days).

- Lose fat and start to reduce the size of fat cells.

- Burn dangerous belly fat.

- Begin to cut diabetes risk by stabilizing blood sugar and boosting insulin sensitivity.

- Begin to improve your heart health by lowering cholesterol and blood pressure.

- Break your addiction to sugar, simple carbohydrates, and junk food.

- Start to feel healthier, stronger, and sexier.

- Feel a sense of mastery that comes from taking control of your health.

- Feel a sense of accomplishment that will fire up your motivation.

- After 14 days on the STAT Plan, you'll transition to the RESTORE Plan.

ARE YOU A SUGAR-HOLIC?

Find out if you are by taking my sugar addiction quiz starting on page 82.

Part of that oath that physicians take when we receive our medical degrees addresses the topic of food—it asks doctors to "apply dietetic measures for the benefit of the sick." Hippocrates, the father of Western medicine, was way ahead of his time in the fifth century BC when he recognized the crucial role that diet played in optimal health and wrote the words, "Let food be thy medicine, and medicine be thy food." Those words have never been truer than they are now, with hundreds of thousands of Americans dying prematurely each year because of the foods they eat.

When patients leave the emergency room, they usually walk out with a handful of prescriptions and appointments for follow-up visits with their doctors. The medical care providers in the ER save lives with STAT treatment, but once the patients are stabilized, they work with their own doctors to figure out a long-term plan to restore their health.

The prescriptions most doctors issue are for medications. But when a doctor medicates problems such as heart disease and diabetes without suggesting major changes to a patient's diet, the patient is missing out on a big part of his or her treatment. In order to really fight these health problems and restore robust health, patients need a different kind of prescription—one that recommends an entirely new way of eating.

I call these recommendations my Doctor's Diet Food Prescriptions.

These Food Prescriptions lay the foundation for all phases of The Doctor's Diet. You can start following them today and let them be your dietary North Star for the rest of your life, both in the active STAT and RESTORE Plans of The Doctor's Diet, and then during the MAINTAIN Plan that will see you through years of your best possible health.

This is just what the ancient doctor, Hippocrates, ordered: an exploration of the specific ways in which food can be your best medicine when it comes to rescuing yourself from diet-related disease. In this part of the book, we'll look at the various components of a healthy diet, and I'll explain the science behind how they help prevent disease and prolong life. I'll also give specific advice about how to make smart choices about these foods and how best to include them in your diet.

PART THREE: RESTORE ROBUST HEALTH WITH THE DOCTOR'S DIET 14-DAY RESTORE PLAN

After you "stop the bleeding" on your unhealthy diet and kick-start dramatic weight loss with the STAT Plan, you'll shift for 14 days to the less-intense RESTORE Plan. On the RESTORE Plan, you will continue to lose weight while enjoying a wider range of foods. If you meet your goal weight during the RESTORE Plan, you'll move on to the MAINTAIN Plan. If not, you'll alternate between STAT and RESTORE until you achieve your goal.

PART FOUR: SAVOR THE REWARDS AS YOU ENJOY EIGHT AMAZING WEIGHT-LOSS PAYOFFS

In this section of the book, I'll tell you *how* all the smart choices you're making with The Doctor's Diet are making you feel better, stronger, sexier, and healthier by extending your life, preventing diseases (including diabetes, cardiovascular disease, arthritis, and some kinds of cancer), boosting your immune system, revving up your mood and your energy, easing your sleep, and even improving the health of your family for generations to come.

PART FIVE: MAINTAIN YOUR WEIGHT LOSS FOR LIFE WITH THE DOCTOR'S DIET MAINTAIN PLAN

Once you've met your weight-loss goal, my MAINTAIN Plan will help you keep the weight off for the rest of your life. The MAINTAIN Plan makes it easy to stay slim with a greater variety of food choices—including many of your favorite foods—and strategies that let you enjoy delicious meals without gaining back all the weight you worked so hard to lose.

We cap off the book with a delicious set of flavorful, easy-to-make recipes that are bursting with fantastic flavor and amazing health benefits. Enjoy fabulous Doctor's Diet versions of chicken parmesan, lasagna, pizza, and more. These recipes, which call for everyday ingredients you may already have on hand, will become your new favorites.

THE DOCTOR'S DIET STRATEGY

✚ Begin with the STAT Plan for the first 14 days.

✚ Move on to the RESTORE Plan for the next 14 days.

✚ Alternate between the STAT Plan and the RESTORE Plan for periods of 14 days each until you meet your weight-loss goal.

✚ Once you have reached your ideal weight, follow the MAINTAIN Plan for permanent weight control.

✚ Use the delicious recipes in my Doctor's Diet Recipe Guide (page 238) for tasty, nutritious meals, or design your own meals according to the Meal Plan Equations for each day.

MOVING TOWARD A BETTER LIFE

With The Doctor's Diet, I focus on how improving your daily eating habits can have a huge impact on your weight and your health. I shine the spotlight on food because, when weight is a health emergency requiring immediate lifestyle treatment, changing your diet is the best place to start. Eating meals with fewer calories and the right combinations of fat-burning foods is the fastest way to kick-start major weight loss.

However, even though a healthy diet is the centerpiece of my program, I do want you to know that exercise is extremely important as well.

All of the changes you are making as part of The Doctor's Diet will be exponentially more successful if you include exercise in your daily life. Every measure of your success—weight loss, lower risk of chronic disease, greater longevity, and improved overall health—will be amplified if you increase your activity levels.

Exercise does amazing things for your body. In addition to helping with weight loss, being active lowers your risk of heart disease, certain cancers, type 2 diabetes, osteoporosis, and depression. It helps strengthen your muscles, improves the health of your organs, boosts your mood, and sharpens your brain. The list of exercise's benefits is almost endless.

A HEALTHY PACE

Because this book focuses on diet, I'm not going to go into detail about training routines, complicated workout strategies, specific exercises, or the many options you can consider when designing a fitness regimen. I don't want to overwhelm you—by following The Doctor's Diet, you're already making so many incredible improvements to your health. Trying to do too much may backfire on you and erode your motivation. I really don't want that to happen!

Right now, taking on the challenge of starting an ambitious new exercise regimen isn't necessary. I do want you to be active, but there's no need to devote hours and hours every week to going to the gym, training for marathons, or becoming a champion mountain biker (although, of course, you're welcome to do that, if you'd like).

My exercise prescription is simple: move your body for at least 30 minutes a day, every day, and try to decrease the amount of time you are sitting throughout the day.

Choose activities you enjoy. Walk, jog, swim, cycle, hit the tread-mill—do whatever you like, as long as you're getting your heart rate up for half an hour a day. When you're ready, try to add in strength training (using weights or your own body weight as resistance) two or three times a week.

But for now, especially if you are just starting out, going for a half-hour walk every day is just right.

If you're very sedentary or obese, the idea of walking half an hour may unnerve you. That's OK—you don't have to start there. Begin with a five-minute walk, if that's what you can comfortably do. Walk five minutes a day during Week One. Then increase it to 10 minutes a day in Week Two. By Week Six, you'll hit your half-hour goal.

As you get fitter and begin to shed pounds, you will feel so good that you'll *want* to move around more. You'll feel stronger, healthier, and more energetic, able to climb stairs without huffing and puffing. You'll find yourself drawn eagerly to more activities, such as gardening, dancing (even if it's by yourself in your living room!), hiking, going for bike rides, or playing with your children or grandchildren.

When all that starts to happen, and you're interested in launching a formal fitness plan, go for it. Or you can just increase the intensity of your daily walks by going farther, faster, or more frequently.

PART ONE
THE DOCTOR'S DIET STAT PLAN

The Doctor's Diet begins with the STAT Plan, which you can start following at your very next meal. The STAT plan is created to give you immediate results. From the moment you bite into your very first STAT Plan meal, you'll be eating meals that are balanced for high-level fat burn and major health benefits.

STAT Plan breakfasts, lunches, dinners, and snacks are designed according to specifically formulated daily Meal Plan Equations, which are created to help jump-start weight loss. They are moderately high in protein, contain smart amounts of unsaturated fat and omega-3 fats, are rich in dietary fiber, and are low in simple carbohydrates and unhealthy fats.

My Meal Plan Equations also give you flexibility. Some of us love big breakfasts and smaller dinners; others prefer eating light in the morning and filling up at lunch or when the mid-afternoon hunger pangs strike. You know your body best, and you know your hungriest times of day. My daily Meal Plan Equations allow you to make choices that will be the most satisfying to you.

For example, in the morning my Meal Plan Equation recommends having a breakfast-sized serving of a high-protein food, such as eggs or yogurt, along with a piece of fruit. If that's all you want, great, but if you like a heartier breakfast, feel free to stir cold cereal into your yogurt, or cook up a bowl of oatmeal, using options from your daily list of Flex-Time Food choices (more on these later). It's a great idea to eat your whole grains early in the day—research suggests that doing so gives you the best bang for your nutritional buck both for weight loss and increased energy—but I'm not going to force any food on you at any time of day! It's up to you.

At lunch, I suggest having a protein for your main dish along with two or more vegetables. If this is plenty for you for your midday meal, that's fine. But if you prefer to have a bit more, feel free to drizzle your vegetables with olive oil or vinaigrette, serve yourself a slice of whole-grain bread, or help yourself to a baked sweet potato using Flex-Time Food choices.

When dinnertime rolls around, my Meal Plan Equation again calls for a protein and some vegetables. Stick with that, or if you have not used up your allotment, use Flex-Time options to add a cup of bean soup or a side of sliced avocado.

As far as snacks are concerned, my Meal Plan Equation offers one snack daily, with lots of choices. For example, you can enjoy a bowl of blueberries and a handful of almonds or sunflower seeds. Or you can choose an apple along with some veggies dipped in hummus or guacamole. If you're someone who does better with two smaller snacks daily, go ahead and use your Flex-Time choices to add a second smaller snack.

FLEX-TIME PUTS YOU IN CHARGE

Flex-Time Foods are an important part of The Doctor's Diet because they help you target your hunger, which boosts your chances of successful weight loss. More importantly, they give you choices, which is something that really matters to me. I don't want anyone telling me exactly what to eat and when to eat it, and I don't think you do, either. That's what fad diets do—but the Doctor's Diet isn't like that. My eating plan isn't about losing a few pounds that you'll gain back next week. It's about making life-saving changes in your eating habits and your weight that will sustain many years of great health. The STAT Plan is designed to meet your needs on a variety of levels. It will start moving you toward dramatic weight loss. It will fuel your body with essential nutrients, while keeping your hunger at bay and ringing the bell on taste and enjoyment. I can't promise you that you'll never feel a single hunger pang on the STAT Plan, but I can tell you that the STAT Plan's formulation of protein, fat, fiber, and complex carbohydrates will leave you feeling surprisingly satisfied even as the pounds start to fall away.

The STAT Plan is lower in daily calories than other parts of The Doctor's Diet. (But don't worry, you won't have to count calories—all you have to do is follow my simple Meal Plan Equations.) Remember, our goal is to "stop the bleeding" on excess weight, and the most effective way to do that is to jump in with both feet and start losing weight.

After two weeks on the STAT Plan, you'll move on to the RESTORE Plan, which offers you even more flexibility.

WHEN SOMEONE IS WHEELED INTO THE ER ON THE EDGE OF DEATH, THE MEDICAL TEAM LEAPS INTO ACTION RIGHT AWAY. THE MEDICAL PHRASE FOR THIS IS "STAT," FROM THE LATIN WORD *STATIM*, WHICH MEANS "IMMEDIATELY".

STAT PLAN GUIDELINES

Before I tell you about the specifics of my daily Meal Plan Equations, here are some basic guidelines for the STAT Plan.

+ **Stay on plan.** For maximum weight loss and the fastest results, follow the STAT Plan as closely as possible. Use daily Meal Plan Equations to create your own daily menus. Or follow my sample 14-day STAT menu, which makes it even easier if you prefer to have your meals designed for you.

+ **Think ahead.** If you have time, sit down each evening and plan your next day's meals. That's the easiest way to make sure you eat the right foods in the right amounts, and that you have everything you need on hand before you start preparing meals. This is something I learned to do a long time ago. It doesn't take long—you can plan your meals in just a couple of minutes. Since it actually ends up saving you time the next day, you come out ahead, time-wise.

+ **Size up your size.** The amount of food we need varies based on our size, as well as age, activity levels, and other factors. When portions are given in a range—for example, three to four ounces of lean meat, poultry or fish—choose the low end of the range if you're smaller (under 5 feet 4 for women or under 5 feet 10 for men), older (over 50), or less active (under 30 minutes daily), and the high end of the range if you're tall, younger, or more active. During the RESTORE and MAINTAIN Plans, active people have even more meal-planning choices.

✦ Get served. Serving sizes really do matter—you can have the healthiest diet in the world, but if you're eating too much of it, you'll never lose weight. For maximum weight loss, stick with suggested serving sizes. In cases where there's a lot of variety in packaged foods—for example, a slice of whole-grain bread can have anything from 40 calories to 140, depending on what's in it and how thickly it's sliced—I will suggest a calorie limit to help you determine the best amount to eat.

✦ Give protein a hand. Meat, poultry, and fish servings are about the same size as the palm of your hand, so feel free to use your palm as a measuring guide for size; the thickness should be similar to that of a deck of playing cards. Measure beans and lentils with a measuring cup.

✦ Choose drinks that accelerate weight loss. Avoid alcoholic beverages, sweetened beverages, or diet sodas. (But don't worry, you'll get to enjoy your favorite "adult" beverages on the RESTORE and MAINTAIN Plans.) For now, enjoy plain water, coffee, green tea, black tea, sparkling water, or water naturally flavored with lemon juice or cucumber slices.

✦ Keep it real. Avoid artificial sweeteners of any kind, because they can reset your brain and cause unnatural sweet cravings. You may use small amounts of honey or light agave nectar syrup (up to a teaspoon a day) to sweeten certain foods.

✦ Fill up with H_2O. Water can help meals feel more filling, so I recommend that you drink an eight-ounce glass of water before each meal and snack (and with your food, if you desire). Drink an additional two to four glasses of water throughout the day.

✦ Scramble it up. Despite the bad press they've gotten over the years (we'll talk more about that later in the book), whole eggs are actually an excellent source of protein and nutrients when eaten in moderation. Enjoy up to seven whole eggs per week (or three per week if you have heart disease or diabetes). Use olive oil cooking spray for scrambling or frying eggs.

✚ **Go low with dairy fat.** Conventional wisdom holds that low-fat and nonfat yogurt and milk are a better choice than full-fat versions. This wisdom is being challenged lately, though, and evidence is adding up to make full-fat dairy less of a villain. We'll go into this in more detail later in the book, but for now I'm going to suggest that in the interest of keeping calories low, stick with low-fat yogurt and milk.

✚ **Spice is nice.** Use healthy fresh or dried seasonings and herbs to liven up your foods: turmeric, curry, basil, oregano, garlic, red pepper flakes, black pepper, and cayenne pepper, to name a few.

✚ **Slip the skip.** It's best not to skip meals, especially breakfast. People who skip meals usually end up eating excessively later in the day.

✚ **Focus on fat-burning fruits.** I recommend you eat two fruits daily as part of the STAT Plan. During the STAT Plan, choose from one medium apple, one cup of fresh or frozen berries, or a grapefruit— compared with other fruits, these are a bit higher in fiber, lower in sugar, and thus better at burning fat. You'll have more fruit choices on the RESTORE and MAINTAIN Plans, but for now, limit yourself to these fat-burning super-fruits.

✚ **Fill 'er up.** Certain vegetables are so low in calories that I call them Anytime Vegetables. They're an important part of lunch, dinner, and snack Meal Plan Equations, but feel free to eat them at breakfast as well, or to munch on them during the day as "free" snacks. Or enjoy my Anytime Vegetable Soup or Anytime Garden Salad whenever you'd like. Find out how to make them in The Doctor's Diet Recipe Guide starting on page 238.

✚ **Get ready for fast results.** Stay on the STAT Plan for 14 days at a time. After that, you'll switch to the RESTORE Plan.

RISE, SHINE, AND EAT

You've heard it a million times: breakfast is the most important meal of the day. But is it really? Instead of filling your tank early in the day, will you lose more weight if you just skip your morning meal?

Here's the deal: Breakfast really is important, and skipping it actually leads to weight gain, not weight loss. Many studies have shown this, including a 2013 study published in the journal *Obesity*. In that study, 50 overweight women were randomly assigned to one of two groups: the big-breakfast group and the big-dinner group.

Both groups ate 1,400 calories worth of food each day. But, as their names suggest, the timing of their eating differed. The big-breakfast group ate a diet that consisted of a breakfast of 700 calories, a lunch of 500 calories, and a dinner of 200 calories. The big-dinner group ate the same foods, but their breakfast and dinner meals (and calories) were switched.

The women in both groups lost significant amounts of weight. But the women in the big-breakfast group lost an average of approximately 19 pounds over the course of 12 weeks, compared to only about 8 pounds in the large dinner group.

Another study, published in 2013 in the journal *Circulation*, found that men who regularly skipped breakfast had a 27 percent higher risk of heart attack or death from coronary heart disease than those who did eat a morning meal. In addition, non-breakfast-eaters in that study reported being hungrier later in the day and ate more food at night.

Other research shows that skipping breakfast raises diabetes risk.

Why the connection between breakfast and heart disease? Researchers think eating breakfast revs up your metabolism early in the morning, paving the way for higher calorie burn all day. Skipping your first meal of the day can lead to obesity, high blood pressure, high cholesterol, and diabetes. So keep my voice in your mind when you're tempted to skip your morning meal (or remember your mom telling you): breakfast is the most important meal of the day!

THE STAT MEAL PLAN EQUATIONS

Use the following Meal Plan Equations to create your daily menus:

STAT BREAKFAST:
1 Breakfast Protein + 1 STAT Fruit

STAT LUNCH:
1 Main-Dish Protein + 2 or more Anytime Vegetables

STAT DINNER:
1 Main-Dish Protein + 2 or more Anytime Vegetables

STAT SNACK:
1 Snack Protein + 1 STAT Fruit + 1 or more Anytime Vegetables

DAILY FLEX-TIME FOODS:
Each day (at the meal or snack of your choice) enjoy these additional foods:

+ 1 Healthy Fat

+ 1 Whole Grain

+ 1 High-Density Vegetable

BREAKFAST PROTEINS

+ 1 medium egg
+ 3 egg whites (separate whites yourself or buy commercially separated whites in a carton)
+ 1 tablespoon nut butter
+ 1 cup plain yogurt (low-fat, regular or Greek)
+ 1 cup milk (dairy or soy, low-fat)
+ Handful (½ ounce) of nuts (almonds, walnuts, peanuts, pecans, pistachios, etc.)
+ Half each of two Breakfast Proteins—for example, half a cup of yogurt with half a handful of nuts

STAT FRUITS

+ 1 medium apple
+ 1 medium grapefruit
+ 1 cup berries (raspberries, strawberries, blueberries, blackberries)

SNACK PROTEINS

+ Handful (½ ounce) of nuts (almonds, walnuts, peanuts, pecans, pistachios, etc.)
+ Handful (½ ounce) of seeds (pumpkin, sunflower, etc.)
+ 1 egg or 3 egg whites
+ 1 tablespoon nut butter
+ 2 tablespoons hummus
+ 1 cup plain yogurt (low-fat, regular or Greek)
+ 1 cup milk (dairy or soy, low-fat)
+ 1 ounce hard cheese (cheddar, Swiss, mozzarella, Parmesan) or feta cheese
+ ½ cup cottage or ricotta cheese (low-fat)
+ Half each of two Snack Proteins—for example, 1 tablespoon hummus and ½ tablespoon nut butter

MAIN-DISH PROTEINS

+ Fish or shellfish (3–4 ounces)
+ Poultry—chicken breast, turkey breast, or lean ground turkey or chicken (3–4 ounces)
+ Lean meat—lean beef, lean ground beef, buffalo meat, ground buffalo meat, pork, lamb, or wild game (3–4 ounces)
+ Tempeh or bean-burger patty (3–4 ounces)
+ Tofu (¾ cup, or 6 ounces)
+ Cooked beans (black, garbanzo/chickpeas, kidney, navy, pinto, soy, white), dried peas, or lentils (½ to ¾ cup)
+ Legume-based soup—lentil (see recipe for my Lentil Soup on page 253), bean, or split pea; up to 2 cups)
+ 2 Breakfast Proteins (for example, a cup of plain yogurt and a handful of nuts)
+ 2 Snack Proteins (for example, 1 ounce hard cheese and one handful of nuts)
+ 1 Breakfast Protein plus 1 Snack Protein (for example, a cup of yogurt and a handful of seeds)
+ 1 Breakfast Protein plus half a Main-Dish Protein (for example, an egg and a cup of bean soup)
+ 1 Snack Protein plus half a Main-Dish Protein (for example, 2 tablespoons of hummus and a 2-ounce chicken breast)
+ Half each of two Main-Dish Proteins (for example, 2 ounces of meat and ¼ cup cooked beans)

ANYTIME VEGETABLES
(Serving size: 1 cup raw leafy greens or ½ cup other vegetables)

+ Anytime Vegetable Soup (see page 257)
+ Anytime Garden Salad (see page 258)
+ Anytime Salsa (see page 258)
+ Alfalfa sprouts
+ Artichoke hearts
+ Artichokes
+ Asparagus
+ Bamboo shoots
+ Beets
+ Bell peppers (red, orange, green, yellow)
+ Bok choy
+ Broccoli
+ Broccoli sprouts
+ Brussels sprouts

- Cabbage
- Carrots
- Cauliflower
- Celery
- Chilies, all types, including jalapeños
- Cilantro
- Collard greens
- Cucumbers
- Eggplant
- Garlic
- Grape leaves
- Green beans
- Green, leafy vegetables (including beet greens, turnip greens, collard greens)
- Jicama
- Kale
- Kelp and other edible seaweeds
- Kohlrabi
- Leeks
- Lettuce, all varieties
- Mesclun
- Mushrooms
- Mustard greens
- Okra
- Onions
- Parsley
- Pea pods
- Pumpkin
- Radishes
- Red cabbage
- Rhubarb
- Romaine lettuce
- Rutabaga
- Salsa made with tomatoes, onions, garlic, and other Anytime Vegetables
- Scallions
- Spinach
- Squash (acorn, butternut, hubbard, summer, winter)
- Swiss chard
- Tomatoes
- Tomato sauce
- Turnip greens
- Turnips
- Vegetable juice
- Watercress
- Yellow wax beans
- Zucchini

HIGH-DENSITY VEGETABLES
(Serving size: ½ cup cooked)

- Corn
- Green lima beans
- Green peas
- Sweet potatoes/yams
- Taro
- Water chestnuts

HEALTHY FATS

+ Olive oil or nut oil (1 tablespoon)
+ Other healthy oils (canola, sesame, soybean, flaxseed, grape seed)
+ Olives (8 black or 10 green, medium-sized)
+ Oil and vinegar dressing or vinaigrette (1½ tablespoons)
+ Avocado (½ small or ⅓ medium)
+ Guacamole (¼ cup), packaged or homemade, with avocado as primary ingredient
+ Handful (½ ounce) of nuts (almonds, walnuts, peanuts, pecans, pistachios, etc.)
+ Handful (½ ounce) of seeds (pumpkin, sunflower, etc.)
+ Nut butter (1 tablespoon)

WHOLE GRAINS

+ Whole-grain bread (1 slice—maximum~100 calories)
+ Whole-grain English muffin (1 whole muffin—maximum~100 calories)
+ Oatmeal—unsweetened (½ cup cooked or 1 ounce dry)
+ Whole-grain cold cereal—whole wheat, oats, or other whole grain listed as first ingredient (1 cup)

Q: I LIKE TO EAT A HEARTY BREAKFAST. CAN I ADD AN EXTRA PROTEIN TO MY MORNING MEAL?

A: Sure you can—flexibility is the name of the game in The Doctor's Diet. Go ahead and choose two breakfast proteins or add a snack protein to your breakfast protein. For instance, you could add nuts to your yogurt or cheese to your egg scramble. But, to keep your daily protein and calorie intake in line, cut back by ½ your protein serving size at lunch or dinner. That way your higher calorie breakfast won't slow down your weight loss.

THE SOY SITUATION

Scientists have gone back and forth about soy foods over the past 20 or so years. After some very positive initial studies, soy was touted as a miracle food with power over multiple diseases and conditions. For example, the plant-based phytoestrogens in soy foods were credited with reducing menopausal hot flashes and reducing the risk of heart disease and some kinds of cancer.

Follow-up research has raised doubts about whether soy is actually as helpful as it first appeared—and whether it's harmful for some people, such as women who have had hormone-positive breast cancer. While we wait to find out more, I suggest you follow your doctor's advice regarding soy foods—if there's a reason your doctor thinks you should avoid them, then I'd go with that advice. If not, my recommendation is to enjoy soy foods in moderation.

Q: WHY IS GRAPEFRUIT RECOMMENDED FOR BREAKFAST IN THE DOCTOR'S DIET?

A: Studies suggest that eating grapefruit has a positive impact on blood sugar, insulin levels, weight loss, and possibly blood pressure. It's packed with nutrients, such as vitamin C, and antioxidants that are believed to reduce the risk of several diseases. There's only one downside to grapefruit: it interferes with the action of certain kinds of drugs, including some benzodiazepines, statins, antihistamines, ulcer drugs, and other medicines. If you are on these or any medication, check with your doctor before making grapefruit a regular part of your diet. If your doc recommends avoiding grapefruit, you can substitute a medium orange instead.

With the STAT Plan, you can choose your own menu using my daily Meal Plan Equations. Or if you prefer, you can use the 14-day menu here. If you do, keep a few things in mind:

Each day's menu includes daily Flex-Time Foods: 1 Whole-Grain, 1 Healthy Fat, and 1 High-Density Vegetable.

Menu items in **bold** have recipes included at the end of this book.

This menu is designed in a traditional breakfast-lunch-dinner style, with soups and salads at lunch and main-dish entrées at dinner. But if you'd like to switch it up, go right ahead—lunch and dinner on the STAT Plan use the same Meal Plan Equations.

G: Whole-Grain Flex-Time Food (1 daily)
F: Healthy Fat Flex-Time Food (1 daily)
V: High-Density Vegetable Flex-Time Food (1 daily)

	BREAKFAST	LUNCH	SNACK	DINNER
	1 Breakfast Protein + 1 STAT Fruit	*1 Main-Dish Protein + 2 or more Anytime Vegetables*	*1 Snack Protein + 1 STAT Fruit + 1 or more Anytime Vegetables*	*1 Main-Dish Protein + 2 or more Anytime Vegetables*
DAY 1	1 grapefruit; **Mediterranean Skillet Scramble (See page 240)**	1 cup **Anytime Vegetable Soup (See page 257);** open-faced grilled chicken breast sandwich (on 1 slice whole-grain toast) (G) with lettuce and sliced tomatoes	Handful of almonds; 1 cup blueberries; sliced carrots	**Shrimp Stir-Fry (See page 268);** ½ cup water chestnuts (V); 1 cup broccoli slaw dressed with **Versatile Vinaigrette** (F) **(See page 244)**
DAY 2	1 cup strawberries; 1 cup yogurt; ½ cup oatmeal (G)	**Greek Lentil Salad (See page 247)**	Handful of pumpkin seeds; 1 apple; 1 cup **Anytime Vegetable Soup (See page 257)**	**Baked Ginger-Marinated Pork (see page 265);** ½ cup baked sweet potato (V); **Garlic-Rosemary Mashed Cauliflower (see page 272)**

	BREAKFAST	LUNCH	SNACK	DINNER
DAY 3	1 apple; 1 cup whole-grain cold cereal (G) with 1 cup milk	**Garbanzo Bean Salad (See page 243)** with **Versatile Vinaigrette (F) (See page 244)**	1 cup strawberries, ½ cup cottage cheese; sliced cucumbers	**Dill Salmon (See page 259);** ½ cup corn (V); sautéed spinach and red peppers
DAY 4	1 grapefruit; 1 hard-boiled egg	Buffalo burger patty with lettuce, sliced tomatoes, onions, pickles, and ½ avocado, sliced (F); whole-grain English muffin (G); 1 cup **Anytime Vegetable Soup (See page 257)**	1 apple; 1 ounce cheddar cheese; sliced red peppers	Grilled chicken breast; ½ cup mashed sweet potatoes (V); garden salad (greens, cherry tomatoes, cucumber, green pepper slices)
DAY 5	1 cup berries; **Spinach Omelet (See page 240)**	**Caesar Salad with Shrimp (See page 249)** and **Garlic Croutons (G) (See page 250)** and Versatile Vinaigrette (F) (See page 244)	Sliced apple spread with 1 tablespoon nut butter; celery sticks	**Beef Skillet Stew (See page 264);** ½ cup green peas (V)
DAY 6	1 apple; ½ cup oatmeal (G) made with water, sprinkled with handful (½ ounce) of nuts	**Beefy Bean and Vegetable Soup (See page 254)** with sliced carrots dipped in ¼ cup guacamole (F)	**Berry Smoothie (See page 238);** sliced cucumbers	**Scallop Kabobs (See page 261);** small ear corn on the cob (V); green beans
DAY 7	1 grapefruit; **Mushroom Omelet (See page 241)** (made with egg whites); 1 slice whole-grain toast (G)	**Quick-Fix Bean Burrito Bowl Salad (See page 251)** with **Versatile Vinaigrette (F) (See page 244)**	1 cup raspberries; 1 cup yogurt; sliced yellow peppers	**Meatza Pizza (See page 263);** garden salad (greens, cherry tomatoes, cucumber, green pepper slices); **Mediterranean Lima Beans** (V) **(See page 274)**
DAY 8	**Berry Smoothie; (See page 238)** ½ cup oatmeal (G) made with water	**Greek Lentil Salad (See page 247)** with 1 cup **Anytime Vegetable Soup (See page 257)**	1 apple; raw veggies dipped in 2 tablespoons hummus and ¼ cup guacamole (F)	**Chicken Stir-Fry (See page 268);** ½ cup water chestnuts (V)

	BREAKFAST	LUNCH	SNACK	DINNER
DAY 9	1 grapefruit; 1 slice whole-grain toast (G) spread with 1 tablespoon nut butter	**Tuscan Bean Salad (See page 247)** with **Versatile Vinaigrette (F) (See page 244)**	1 cup blackberries; handful of peanuts; raw broccoli florets	Grilled sirloin steak; **Baked Sweet Potato Fries** (V) **(See page 275); Roasted Eggplant (See page 272)**
DAY 10	**Veggie Smoothie (See page 239)**; ½ cup oatmeal (G) made with water	**Chef Salad (See page 250)** with **Versatile Vinaigrette** (F) **(See page 244)**	1 grapefruit; handful of sunflower seeds; celery sticks	**Grilled Portobello Mushrooms (See page 270)**; ½ cup green peas (V)
DAY 11	1 cup berries; ½ cup oatmeal (G) made with water, 1 cup plain yogurt	Sliced roast beef; raw veggies with ½ cup fresh salsa and ¼ cup guacamole (F)	Handful of almonds; 1 cup blueberries; sliced carrots	**Lemon-Rosemary Salmon (See page 259)**; small ear corn on the cob (V)
DAY 12	1 grapefruit; scrambled eggs (made with 1 egg or 3 egg whites); 1 slice whole-grain toast (G)	**Minestrone Soup (See page 254); Anytime Garden Salad (See page 258)** with **Versatile Vinaigrette** (F) **(See page 244)**	1 apple; 1 ounce cheddar cheese; sliced yellow peppers	**Veggie Stir-Fry with Cashews (See page 269)**; ½ cup green peas (V)
DAY 13	**High-Protein Breakfast Smoothie (See page 239)** (G)	**Old West Chili (See page 256)** with sliced tomatoes	1 cup raspberries; 1 cup yogurt; sliced cucumbers dipped in ¼ cup guacamole (F)	1 cup **Anytime Vegetable Soup (See page 257); Salsa Chicken (See page 266)** served over ½ cup baked mashed sweet potatoes (V)
DAY 14	1 apple spread with 1 tablespoon nut butter; ½ cup oatmeal (G) made with water	**Caprese Salad (See page 248)** with **Versatile Vinaigrette** (F) **(See page 244)**	**Veggie Smoothie (See page 239)**	**Garlic Shrimp (See page 261)**; ½ cup green lima beans (V)

PART TWO
LIFE-SAVING FOOD PRESCRIPTIONS

"Let food be thy medicine, and medicine be thy food." -Hippocrates

When patients are brought into the emergency room suffering from a heart attack, stroke, or other life-threatening emergency, doctors and nurses jump into action, administering treatment and giving medications in hopes of pulling them from the jaws of death.

Once they're stabilized—once we "stop the bleeding," so to speak—our emergency room patients go back to their own doctors and specialists, who work with them to make changes that will keep them out of the ER in the future.

After leaving the ER, patients typically receive a stack of prescriptions. Post–heart attack, for example, they might walk out with prescriptions for blood thinners, beta-blockers, or statins.

Now that you've started The Doctor's Diet, and you're at least a few meals into the STAT Plan—now that you're taking crucial steps to stabilize your own weight emergency—I'm going to follow my typical ER procedure and hand you a stack of prescriptions.

Unlike what you'd get after an ER visit, though, these aren't prescriptions for medicines. They're prescriptions for food.

My Doctor's Diet Food Prescriptions will help you not only lose weight, but aid you in restoring your vitality and lowering your risk of disease. They'll explain in detail the science behind the design of The Doctor's Diet, why certain foods can boost your health, and why other foods can devastate it. They'll give you a step-by-step blueprint for healthy eating—and it's one that you can follow for the rest of your life.

Sure, you could just follow the meal plans in this book and lose weight without understanding the "why" behind the recommendations I make. But I don't think that's the best way to go. Unless you really get the thinking behind my dietary advice, you won't really own it yourself.

I'm a big believer in everyone owning their own health-care decisions. And I'm a big believer in the power of "why."

Here's the way I look at it. If someone suggests that I do something, and they tell me *why* I ought to do it, I'm much more likely to understand it and to want to do it that way than I am if I don't get an explanation. (We're also more likely to remember to do something a certain way if we understand why we're doing it.) When I was in medical school, and one of my professors demonstrated a particular way to suture a laceration, I picked it up a whole lot quicker when I understood the *why* of it, rather than just the *how*. For example, the kind of suture that is best for a deep wound may leave too much of a scar if it's used on a superficial skin wound.

That's why I want you to understand not just *which* foods are best for your health, but *why* they are so good.

I don't want you choosing one food over another because you're thinking, "That's what Dr. Travis thinks I should eat." It's not about me—it's about you, your body, and your health. When you understand how food impacts your blood, your organs, and every cell in your body, making the healthiest choices becomes easier. When you own your decisions, you're better able to live them.

CONTRADICTORY RESEARCH— WHAT SHOULD YOU BELIEVE?

Before we go any further, let's talk a little about the scientific research behind my recommendations.

Sometimes it seems like nutrition scientists are purposely trying to confuse us. Foods are like celebrities: overnight, they go from being stars to pariahs. One day we hear that a certain food will cure whatever ails us; the next day we are told that the very same food will kill us. Well, which is it? What's going on here? If the scientists and doctors aren't even sure whether to eat some of these foods, how are people without nutritional and medical training supposed to decide what to eat?

Listen, I'll be completely honest with you. I'm a doctor with an avid interest in nutrition—I make a point of staying on top of all the latest research—and even I struggle with this conundrum in my own life nearly every day. Not long ago, I read a study saying people should stay away from corn, for example. The very next day I read a different study that said corn is great! So which is it? Honestly, it leaves me standing in front of the refrigerator some days not knowing what the heck to eat!

That's why, even with the Food Prescriptions in The Doctor's Diet, you shouldn't go overboard with any one food. With the corn example, my position is that until the studies on corn become clearer, I'll go ahead and have an occasional ear of corn (because I enjoy corn on the cob, especially in the summer), but until there's more clarity on the question of how good it is for me, I only eat corn now and then.

My advice is to always be moderate, and be sure to mix things up. Even when the research is heavily in favor of a certain food, it doesn't make sense to get obsessed with it. Legumes are great, but that doesn't mean you should eat only lentils for breakfast, lunch, and dinner every day of your life. It's not ideal to eat too much of any single food, even if researchers are calling it a "superfood."

Go for variety—have lentils in your soup today, black beans in your burrito tomorrow, kidney beans in your salad the next day. Enjoy corn on the cob at your next barbecue, but don't put it on the menu every single meal. Optimal health comes from eating a variety of healthful foods, not expecting one food to be a nutritional knight in shining armor that will fix all the health problems in your life.

MY FOOD PRESCRIPTIONS

In the following section of the book, I'll give you my 10 Food Prescriptions for optimal health. They are the backbone of The Doctor's Diet. Read them as you work your way through the 14-day STAT Plan. Then, by the time you're ready to begin the RESTORE Plan, you'll have all the knowledge you need to own your new eating choices for the rest of your life.

We've all done it: eaten something so fast that we don't even taste it. We've inhaled bags of chips, sucked down giant milkshakes, mowed through a plate of cookies, and swallowed a candy bar so fast that we don't even remember unwrapping it.

We do it when we're eating on the run, grabbing something quick—usually a greasy burger or a sweet dessert—and stuffing it into our mouths so quickly that it barely registers in our mind that we're eating.

We do it at home, plowing through our favorite snack foods while we're watching television after a long day.

We even do it at mealtimes, when we're sitting down to the same old thing, mindlessly shoveling food into our mouths as we sort through the mail, read the newspaper, or check in with friends on Facebook.

You probably did it at your most recent meal. Quick: What did you have for dinner last night? If you can't remember, it's probably because you wolfed it down mindlessly.

If you're anything like me, you can mindlessly inhale a big bowl of ice cream and be hard pressed to remember, even half an hour later, what kind of ice cream it was. This kind of eating is called mindless eating because while our mouths do the chewing, our minds are paying zero attention to what we eat. When we eat mindlessly, we don't taste our food or appreciate the flavors of what we're consuming. What's worse, we don't pay attention to how much we're eating, or what ingredients are in the food we're gobbling up. We ignore the signals our body sends when we start to feel full. We just keep eating and eating, making poor choices, focusing on everything else except our body's reactions to the food we're taking in.

WHEN WE EAT MINDLESSLY, WE DON'T TASTE OUR FOOD OR APPRECIATE THE FLAVORS OF WHAT WE'RE CONSUMING. WE DON'T PAY ATTENTION TO WHAT OR HOW MUCH WE'RE EATING, AND WE IGNORE THE SIGNALS OUR BODY SENDS WHEN WE START TO FEEL FULL.

I think mindless eating is one of the top contributors to America's obesity epidemic. I know there's a lot more to it—we eat too much, we eat the wrong kinds of food. But have you ever thought about why we do that? Nobody's setting out to gain excess weight. Nobody intentionally eats foods that will put them on the fast track to the emergency room.

We don't sit down at the dinner table and say to ourselves, "I am going to eat so much at this meal that my pants won't button an hour from now." We don't grab a bottle of cola and think, "What my body really needs right now is 16 teaspoons of sugar and a load of artificial caramel color!" And we certainly don't wish, when we're biting into a piece of coffee cake, "I sure hope this raises my heart disease risk!"

This is the problem: we are so accustomed to not thinking about the food we eat that we've eaten ourselves sick. Eating mindlessly gets us nowhere but to the ER and an early grave.

It's time to change all that and start eating *mindfully*. It's time to start paying attention—really paying attention—to what you put in your mouth, how it tastes, how it makes your body feel, what it's made of, and what potential it has to save or sabotage your health.

It's time to start listening to your body while you eat, so when it starts telling you that it's getting full, you'll hear its message loud and clear and put down your fork.

It's time to bring mindfulness—an ancient principle of awareness, awakening, and enlightenment espoused by philosophers and wise people throughout history—to your kitchen table.

IF YOU CAN'T REMEMBER WHAT FOOD YOU HAD AT YOUR LAST MEAL, YOU PROBABLY ATE IT MINDLESSLY, WITHOUT THINKING OR NOTICING HOW IT TASTED OR HOW YOUR BODY REACTED TO IT.

My 10 Food Prescriptions are all really important, but being mindful of what you eat is the most important one of all. Mindful eating is my number one Food Prescription, because if you can open your mind and become fully aware of food and its impact on your health and your life, everything else you do as you follow The Doctor's Diet will be easier. In and of itself, that one change alone could make all the difference for you in your quest to lose weight for good.

OPENING YOUR MIND'S EYE

Mindfulness is the process of being aware—intensely aware of everything going on around you. Philosophers, such as the Buddha, taught their followers to use mindfulness to achieve spiritual enlightenment. I'm no philosopher, and I'm certainly not going to try to tell you how to run your spiritual life. But as a doctor I've learned that mindfulness plays a crucial role in good health.

When you're mindful, you become more aware of the options you have, and you fully understand and accept that the decisions you make influence your health and well-being. In my experience, mindful choices are the best kind of choices, because they are based on knowledge and clear-eyed thought, rather than ignorance and uninformed assumptions.

FULLY CONSCIOUS EATING

So, what is mindful eating? Here's a great way of thinking about it. You know *Highlights*, the children's magazine that you see in dentists' offices? One of the regular features in *Highlights* was a comic strip about two characters, Goofus and Gallant. The strip showed how Goofus and Gallant acted completely different in various social situations. For example, on a crowded bus, Goofus would stay seated while an elderly woman held on to a pole for dear life; Gallant would get up and offer her his seat. Goofus would keep the dollar he found on the street; Gallant would put up a sign looking for the money's owner. You get the idea.

You can apply Goofus and Gallant thinking to mindful eating as well. In most eating-related situations, there are mindless choices and mindful choices. For example:

✢ **Reading labels.** Mindless eaters ignore them, paying no attention to a food's ingredients. Mindful eaters read them carefully, using the information on them to pick healthy foods and limit those with added sugar, unhealthy fats, and artificial ingredients.

✢ **Choosing portion sizes.** Mindless eaters guess at them and overeat. Mindful eaters take note of serving sizes on nutrition labels and help themselves to a limited amount of food by using measuring spoons, cups, a scale, or a memory device (such as, a serving of protein is about the size of the palm of your hand, minus your fingers).

✢ **Grocery shopping.** Mindless eaters wander up and down the aisles buying whatever captures their interest. Mindful eaters make a list and stick with it.

✢ **Meal planning.** Mindless eaters wait until mealtime to figure out what to make. Mindful eaters plan meals in advance, either by the day or week, making sure they have all the right foods on hand for healthy meals.

✢ **Choosing foods.** Mindless eaters eat with only the present moment in mind; if something looks good, they consume it. Mindful eaters consider food choices before rushing to eat, considering whether the food fits in with their short-term and long-term health goals.

✢ **Eating.** Mindless eaters watch TV, read, stand, walk around, drive, talk on the phone, or do many other kinds of multitasking while eating. Mindful eaters focus on their food, blocking out other distractions so they can taste, smell, and enjoy what they're eating.

✢ **Timing.** Mindless eaters rush through their meals. Mindful eaters slow down, allowing themselves to taste every bite, to chew their food fully, and to give their bodies time to recognize and react to food.

✢ **Tasting.** Mindless eaters barely notice the taste of foods. Mindful eaters savor every bite, paying attention to flavor, texture, spiciness, crunch, chewiness, and other attributes of deliciousness.

✦ **Appreciating natural flavor.** Mindless eaters sprinkle salt or sugar on everything. Mindful eaters reduce their dependence on salt and sugar and enjoy the natural sweet and savory flavors of food.

✦ **Focusing on the body's reaction to food.** Mindless eaters ignore feelings of hunger and fullness. Mindful eaters listen to the signals sent to their brain by their digestive system and respect the body's innate ability to recognize hunger and satiety. (This is a skill that may take a while to develop, so don't worry if at first you're not good at deciphering these signals.)

GETTING TO KNOW HUNGER

If you've been eating mindlessly for years—or even decades—you may be very much out of touch with what hunger and satiety feel like. Eating mindfully starts with getting reacquainted with these feelings. One way to do this is to let yourself get hungry, and to pay attention to how it feels. As an experiment, go a little longer than usual without eating, and then spend a few minutes focusing on your sensations. Sit in a quiet room, without any distractions, and really zone in on what your body is telling you. Mindfully experience the feeling of an empty stomach, the "growling" of your belly, the sense of emptiness or gnawing that occupies your middle. Do a mental body scan to look for other signs of hunger. Do you feel headachey at all? Are you light-headed? Do you feel impatient or irritable? These sensations can be unpleasant, but they are true signs of physical hunger, and it's good to be in touch with them so you can recognize them.

Then, go into the kitchen and eat a meal. (The best time to do this is when you're alone, so you can really zero in on your physical responses.) Eat slowly, keeping close track of how you feel. Notice your stomach feeling fuller and the emptiness in your belly subsiding. Note any changes you experience in your body and mind as you move from hunger to satiety.

During the days that follow, continue to monitor these feelings. Over time, you'll get much better at recognizing them, and at distinguishing hunger from thirst and fatigue, as well as from emotional hungers such as boredom, sadness, and loneliness.

Here's another reason why developing the skill of mindful eating will help you lose weight. As you start to follow The Doctor's Diet and begin to implement all of my Food Prescriptions, you'll be eating food in a much more natural form than you may be used to. As you cut out added sugar, unhealthy fats, fried foods, preserved meats, and other kinds of processed foods, you'll replace them with whole, unprocessed foods, such as vegetables, fruits, nuts, legumes, whole grains, and lean meats and fish.

At first this change may be jarring to your taste buds—food may taste dull and boring without all those additives, sugars, and fake flavorings. But be patient—I promise you that before you know it, your taste buds will come around to your new way of eating, and your palate will be reset. Real foods may taste a bit bland at first compared with fake foods, but by cutting down on processed foods and using mindfulness to fully taste and appreciate whole foods, you'll soon come to prefer their natural flavors.

Resetting your palate is a crucial part of The Doctor's Diet. Once you do this, you'll be much better able to appreciate subtle flavors, and you will no longer need a big wallop of sugar or a heavy shake of salt to make foods taste good.

FOLLOWING THE DOCTOR'S DIET RESETS YOUR PALATE SO YOU CAN TRULY ENJOY THE TASTES OF WHOLE, NATURAL FOODS.

OPEN YOUR EYES TO BLIND EATING

Mindfulness means more than being aware of what you're eating—it's being fully conscious of what is in the food you eat and being honest with yourself about its potential impact on your health.

The opposite of mindful eating is blind eating—for example, the kind of eating you do in restaurants when you pretend that the 12-ounce steak you ordered is really just 3 ounces, or when you tell yourself that the battered fried fish is really just as good a choice as a filet grilled without coating.

We sometimes deceive ourselves about food, telling ourselves lies about the choices we make. Our bodies know the truth, though.

Mindful eating means being honest with yourself about serving sizes, ingredients, and choices. It means owning your decisions and making them based on facts, not fallacies. When you're ordering fish at a restaurant, find out how it's cooked. Quiz your server about whether it's breaded and fried. Ask if it can be cooked "naked"—grilled or baked without any extra fats or breading.

Once you know the facts and make a selection about what you're going to eat, own that decision 100 percent! If you go with baked fish, enjoy it and give yourself credit for choosing wisely (but celebrate with a pat on the back, not a piece of cherry cheesecake!). And if you opt for the breaded fish, own that decision as well—don't blame it on someone else, or tell yourself little stories that it was your only choice, or play dumb with yourself and believe that all that fried breading doesn't really make a difference to your health. It does, and when you decide to have it, you need to own that choice as something you did with your nutritional eyes wide open.

It's all up to you—you have the choice at every meal, every snack, to eat in a way that contributes to weight loss and robust health.

TRY IT: PRACTICE EATING MINDFULLY

After a lifetime of mindless eating, eating mindfully takes some practice. Here's a really easy way to get started. Take a small square (about half an ounce) of really amazing, intense dark chocolate (at least 70 percent cocoa). Sit in a quiet, distraction-free place and eat it in a mindful, focused, attentive way.

As you unwrap it, notice everything about the experience—the crinkly sound of the foil wrapper, the earthy aroma of cocoa, the color and smoothness of the chocolate in your fingers, the feeling of your taste buds releasing saliva.

Place half the chocolate square on your tongue, and notice how it feels. Allow it to melt in your mouth without chewing it.

Taste the chocolate's creamy richness as it softens. Identify the flavors you notice—sweetness, bitterness, vanilla, spiciness; even a note of mocha or citrus may play out on your tongue.

Slowly start to chew the square and see how the taste changes. Notice how your body is reacting to it. Is your mouth watering? Are you feeling a sense of pleasure? What are all of your senses reporting to you about the chocolate? Swallow that piece, sit for a moment reflecting on the experience, and then have the other piece. As you do, pay attention to every one of your senses and note how the second piece may taste different than the first. Over time you won't find yourself missing all the added sugar of milk chocolate and you'll learn to appreciate the richness of darker chocolate (and the added health benefit).

This exercise works well with any food—sweet-tart apples, creamy yogurt, tangy kale, or crunchy almonds. Your goal is to practice being fully aware of how the food tastes and how your body and senses react to it. As you become more aware, you'll start to notice that foods satisfy you in a whole new way. A tiny piece of chocolate eaten mindfully can be way more enjoyable than an entire candy bar inattentively gobbled up.

Mindfulness is like a muscle—the more you work it, the stronger it gets. Practice it at every meal and snack, and its benefits will start to flow. As you become more mindful, you may discover that the foods you like taste even better. You may also find that whole, natural foods you once thought of as bland are actually bursting with flavor.

IT'S NOT A RACE!

How many times have you spent hours cooking a meal and then just a few minutes eating it? Or, if you're not a cook, how many times have you snarfed down a meal that someone else spent a long time creating? Instead of eating slowly, savoring your (or your favorite cook's) hard work, and relishing the flavors in your food, you chomp it all down at breakneck speed.

Your food will taste better and be more satisfying if you slow down while you eat it—that's another part of mindfulness. When you eat at a leisurely pace, you give yourself time to taste and enjoy your food.

Slowing down doesn't just increase the pleasure of eating. It actually impacts the amount of food you eat.

Your digestive system and your brain communicate via hormones such as leptin and ghrelin. Hormones tell you when you're hungry and signal you when you're full. But hormones sometimes take a while to act.

If you're eating rapidly and mindlessly, by the time your brain gets the message that you're not hungry anymore, you may already have consumed way more food than you actually need.

If you're eating slowly and mindfully, your hormones have time to do their job properly. When you've had enough to eat, they can get the message out to you, and you can stop eating before taking in a whole lot of extra calories.

A CURE FOR PORTION DISTORTION

Eating mindfully extends beyond the awareness of what you eat and whether it benefits your health. In order to succeed at weight loss, you have to pay attention to how much you eat.

Even if you eat all of the super-healthy foods I recommend and stay away from all junk food, you won't shed pounds and burn excess fat unless you cut back on calories. It's a simple equation: When you eat more calories than you burn, you gain weight. When you eat fewer calories than you burn, you lose weight.

It's not exactly a "calories in, calories out" situation. Some foods contribute more to weight loss than others. For example, research suggests that when you eat 100 calories worth of nuts, some 10 or 15 of those calories go through your body undigested.

But in general, the only way you're going to lose weight is by taking in fewer calories than you've become accustomed to. To do this, you have to be totally mindful of how much you're eating. You have to commit fully to becoming an expert in portion sizes.

You can't count on eyeballing portion sizes. For one thing, we are absolutely terrible at approximating how much food we eat. Even if a piece of steak looks like it weighs three ounces, it's likely to be four, five, or six ounces—or more. A half cup of ice cream is likely to be closer to half a pint. And in the opposite direction, what looks like two cups of salad greens may be more like a cup or a cup and a half.

Go ahead and blame all this portion distortion on the fact that food has gotten so much bigger in the past two decades. When I was a kid, foods like bagels, muffins, pizza slices, sodas, cookies, and even ice cream cones were way smaller than they are now—and I'm not that old, so it's not like I'm dredging up memories from the Great Depression. A bagel that you buy in a bakery or grocery store today may actually contain as many as four servings of bread. Take a look at a bag of mini bagels in the grocery store and you'll see that, rather than being tiny little things that many of us could easily eat two or three of, these "mini" bagels actually weigh in at about an ounce—which is equal to one serving of bread.

Muffins are worse. I've seen muffins that are so big a bodybuilder would have trouble lifting them. These are muffins that weigh in with more calories and fat than two candy bars.

Like it or not, in order to lose weight you have to get real about portion sizes. You have to be mindful of how much you *should* be eating, and how much you *are* eating. To do this you've got to use some kind of measuring system.

I don't care what you use to gauge your portion sizes. You can weigh it on a scale or measure it with a cup or spoon. You can learn how much your kitchen dishes hold—that way, you know when you have cereal in the blue flowered bowl that you should pour in just enough to reach the third leaf under the rim. You can go by the sizes of your hands or fingers—for example, an ounce of cheese is about the size of your thumb, a medium apple or orange is about the size of your fist, and a serving of nuts is about a handful. You can even count your foods—for example, with the peanuts I buy, a one-ounce serving is just about 40 nuts.

And of course, keep an eye on food labels—they tell you exactly what you're getting.

Whatever you do, just make sure you're being honest with yourself. If you fill your hand with 60 nuts and call it 40, you're getting 50 percent more calories. The only one you cheat is yourself.

MINDFUL SNACKING

Allowing yourself to get ravenously hungry between meals is a recipe for dietary disaster. That's why the STAT Plan includes one snack daily, which you can eat whenever you need it: mid-morning, mid-afternoon, or after dinner.

Eating small, healthy, well-constructed snacks between meals can boost your energy, make it easier for you to stick with your eating plan, and contribute to your daily requirements for fiber, protein, vitamins, and other important nutrients.

Careful snacking can also help keep blood sugar levels stable, which heads off the kind of binging that can occur when you're very hungry.

The key to smart snacking is making mindful choices. Having a snack doesn't mean eating cookies, ice cream, cake, or a bag of chips. It means enjoying sensible-size portions of healthy foods.

The most effective snacks usually combine complex carbohydrates with lean protein. This combo gives you an immediate energy fix and puts some fuel in your tank for later on, too. Together, protein and complex carbohydrates fill you up and help chase hunger pangs away.

KEEP IT ALL IN MIND

As you move on through the rest of my Food Prescriptions, remember to keep your mind as open as possible. Be aware not only of what and how you're eating, but of foods you may have turned away from in the past that might be worth reconsidering.

Opening yourself to a full awareness of food's impact on your life and health will make it easier for you to make choices that will pay off now and in the future. If you really, truly set your mind to it, permanent weight loss is within your reach.

By now you've probably noticed that protein is an important part of The Doctor's Diet. All of the meals and snacks in the STAT Plan, the RESTORE Plan, and the MAINTAIN Plan contain protein. There's a really good reason for this: protein is an incredibly effective weight-loss tool—provided you know how to use it.

When it comes to losing weight, protein has power, and The Doctor's Diet is designed to harness that power.

What do I mean when I talk about putting protein to work for you? I'm referring to the fact that protein is most beneficial to your weight-loss efforts if you include it in your diet in a balanced, strategic way. You can't just binge on meat, eggs, and other high-protein foods whenever you feel like it—that won't lead to better health.

It all comes down to balance. You can get the most weight-control bang from your protein buck by making sure you're eating balanced amounts of protein and the right kinds of protein foods, and that you're timing them in the most effective way possible throughout your day.

Here's an example of what I mean. I've already talked about the importance of eating a good breakfast, but there's even more to the story than that. It's not just *whether* you eat breakfast that matters. The protein content of your first meal of the day also makes a big difference.

In a 2013 study published in the *American Journal of Clinical Nutrition*, researchers looked at the effect of a high-protein breakfast on hunger and snacking. Some of the subjects ate a protein-rich breakfast (35 grams of protein, 350 calories), some ate a moderate amount of protein with their morning meal (13 grams, 350 calories), and some had no protein (or any other nutrients, for that matter, because they skipped breakfast completely). The high-protein and moderate-protein meals had the same amount of fat, fiber, sugar, and calories.

Having a protein-rich breakfast really paid off. Researchers found that compared with the others, the higher-protein breakfast group reported feeling more satiated and less hungry throughout the day, and experienced fewer food cravings. They also reduced their evening snacking on high-sugar, high-fat foods—evidence that eating a high-protein breakfast pays off throughout the day.

Other studies have found that people lose more weight and keep it off more effectively when they include protein in each meal and snack—which is exactly what The Doctor's Diet does.

SCRAMBLED ADVICE

For years we've been told to avoid eggs because of their cholesterol. But it turns out this may not be necessary. For people without heart disease, diabetes, or high cholesterol, eating an egg a day appears to have no negative impact on heart health.

It's true that egg yolks contain a fair amount of cholesterol. But they're also good sources of protein, several B vitamins, choline, vitamin D, and vitamin E. Depending on how the chickens who laid them are fed, eggs can also be a good source of omega-3 fatty acids and lutein, which helps with eye health.

I love eggs not only because of their nutrients. For someone like me who is not a natural vegetable lover, eggs are a fantastic veggie-delivery vehicle. I'm not crazy about most raw veggies, but I eat them up when they're hidden in an omelet made with a mix of whole eggs and egg whites.

Choose eggs from hens fed an antibiotic-free vegetarian diet. Limit yourself to one yolk a day, or three per week if you have heart disease or diabetes. We don't know exactly why, but in studies of groups of people with diabetes, those who limit egg intake seem to have less heart disease. We need more research to understand the connection—or whether there really is one—but in the meantime, we'll go with that advice because it's the best we have.

THE POWER BEHIND PROTEIN

Full disclosure: we don't know exactly why protein helps with weight loss. One reason is that it has an impact on the action of ghrelin, known as the "hunger hormone," and leptin, the "satiety hormone"—which is why people who eat protein at each meal find they feel fuller and less hungry during the hours after they eat than do people who skimp on protein. In fact, protein is more satiating than fat or carbohydrates.

Another explanation for protein's contribution to weight loss is its ability to help keep blood sugar levels stable. When you eat a low-protein, high-carbohydrate meal, your blood sugar soars soon after you eat. What goes up must come down, and it doesn't take long for blood sugar that shoots up quickly to come falling down fast, too. When blood sugar comes down fast, alarms go off in your endocrine system. Hormones tell your brain that you need more food in order to get blood sugar levels back up, and before you know it, you're wandering around the kitchen looking for a snack just a short time after you finished your meal.

Something different happens when you eat a protein-rich meal. Instead of skyrocketing, your blood sugar levels go up gradually, allowing your endocrine system to proceed at a normal pace as it does its job of getting energy to all of your body's cells. Without a dramatic spike, there's no dramatic fall, meaning no sudden hormone alerts telling you to eat something right away, meaning no sudden, intense desires to inhale jelly donuts or chocolate cake.

Without those blood sugar spikes and constant cravings, you're much better able to make it to your next meal without wanting to fill your tank with lots of extra food.

PROTEIN'S OTHER PROMISES

Eating a protein-rich diet has other benefits as well:

+ **Protein vs. paunch.** Protein helps burn belly fat. In studies, people who eat higher-protein diets lose more belly fat than those who eat lower-protein diets with similar calorie counts.

+ **Muscle maker.** Protein helps preserve muscle. When you're losing weight, you take in fewer calories than you need, which forces your body to burn fat for fuel. When you eat a high-carbohydrate diet, your body is more likely to turn to muscles for stored fuel rather than fat. But eating a protein-rich diet protects your muscles and pushes your body to rely on fat rather than your hard-earned muscles.

+ **Speedier healing.** Protein is a necessary nutrient that just about every part of your body needs. Protein contributes to the growth, development, and healthy function of each cell in your skin, muscles, organs, and glands. It also allows your immune system to work effectively.

+ **Tool for the ticker.** Your heart benefits from protein as well. Eating a diet rich in lean protein—I'm not talking fatty steaks and processed lunch meats here, but lean, healthy protein sources—benefits your blood cholesterol levels.

EATING FROM THE SEA

One of the absolute best sources of protein is seafood—especially fish and shellfish that contain omega-3 fatty acids, a type of polyunsaturated fat that has a wide range of health benefits. Omega-3s are credited with reducing heart disease risk, boosting brain health, and supporting eye health, and studies are under way to tease out other benefits as well.

Nearly all fish contain omega-3s, but some have especially high levels, such as herring, salmon (farmed and wild), mackerel, tuna (bluefin has the most, followed by canned white and light), sardines, swordfish, and trout (and oysters and mussels in the mollusk department). In order to get the omega-3 fatty acids you need, I recommend including at least eight ounces of omega-3-rich fish in your diet each week.

The only downside of eating seafood is that nearly all fish and shellfish contain some amount of mercury, a toxic metal. For nonpregnant adults, eating moderate amounts of most kinds of seafood usually poses little health risk. However, too much mercury can more easily harm the nervous system of an unborn baby or a young child.

To limit the risk from mercury, the US Food and Drug Administration advises women who may become pregnant, pregnant women, nursing mothers, and young children to:

+ Avoid types of fish that are typically high in mercury—including shark, swordfish, tilefish, and king mackerel.

+ Limit intake of lower-mercury fish to 12 ounces per week. Some of the most commonly eaten lower-mercury seafood includes shrimp, canned light tuna, salmon, pollock, and catfish.

- Limit intake of canned albacore (white tuna), which has more mercury than light tuna, to 6 ounces per week.

- Check local advisories about the safety of fish caught by family and friends in local lakes, rivers, and coastal areas. (Yes, even freshwater fish can contain traces of mercury.) If no advice is available, eat up to 6 ounces per week of fish caught in local waters, but don't consume any other fish during that week.

Check out the National Resources Defense Council's guide to mercury in fish at the following link: http://www.nrdc.org/health/effects/mercury/guide.asp. You can also download a cool app from the Monterey Bay Aquarium called "Seafood Watch": http://www.montereybayaquarium.org/cr/cr_seafoodwatch/sfw_aboutsfw.aspx.

HOW MUCH PROTEIN SHOULD YOU EAT?

In The Doctor's Diet, up to a third of your daily calories come from the protein in meat, poultry, seafood, beans and peas, eggs, dairy, nuts, and seeds. That balanced amount gives you all of protein's benefits while leaving room in your diet for all the other nutrient-rich foods you need, including healthy fats and complex carbohydrates.

Some diets call for even more protein than that, but as far as I'm concerned, they're on the wrong track. The weight-loss benefits of protein level off at 30 to 35 percent. There's simply no benefit to super-high-protein diets, especially because they tend to be very low in fruits, vegetables, whole grains, and all the other life-supporting foods that can help us stay healthy.

Excess protein can also put a strain on your kidneys, although that's usually only a problem for people who have kidney disease or other health problems related to protein metabolism.

PROTEIN IN FOOD

PROTEIN SOURCE	GRAMS OF PROTEIN
1 cup milk	8
1 cup soy milk	6-8
1 large egg	6
1 large egg white	4
½ cup low-fat cottage cheese	12-15
3 ounces canned tuna, drained	22
1 ounce peanuts	7
1 ounce almonds	6
2 tablespoons peanut butter	7
1 ounce cheddar cheese	7
3 ounces meat	21
8 ounces plain, low-fat yogurt	14
½ cup cooked beans (black, kidney, etc.)	7-8
½ cup cooked lentils	9
½ cup chickpeas	6
¼ cup hummus	5
1 cup unsweetened almond milk	1
1 ounce frozen edamame	3
3 ounces roasted chicken or turkey breast meat	24-27
3 ounces sirloin steak	25
3 ounces cooked salmon	18-21
3 ounces tofu	6-13

WHAT ABOUT RED MEAT?

Although it's fine to include some lean beef, pork, and lamb in your diet, you're better off relying mostly on poultry, fish, dairy, nuts, and legumes to meet the lion's share of your protein needs.

Various studies have found that people who eat a lot of meat tend to be less healthy than those who eat less meat. For example, in a Harvard study published in 2012 in the *Archives of Internal Medicine*, researchers found that red meat consumption was associated with an increased risk of death from heart disease, cancer, and other causes. The study also showed that substituting other healthy protein sources, such as fish, poultry, nuts, and legumes, was associated with lower risk of potentially fatal diseases.

The study, which followed 120,000 men and women for 28 years, found that one daily serving of unprocessed red meat (about the size of a deck of cards) was associated with a 13 percent increased risk of mortality during the study period, and one daily serving of processed red meat (one hot dog or two slices of bacon) was associated with a 20 percent increased risk.

Other studies have found connections between red meat consumption and type 2 diabetes.

What's behind all this? According to the researchers, red meat, especially processed meat, contains ingredients that have been linked to increased risk of chronic diseases, such as cardiovascular disease and cancer. These include iron (specifically, a type called "heme" iron), saturated fat, sodium, nitrites, and certain carcinogens that are formed during cooking.

But hold on—there may be much more to it than that.

The question of whether red meat is "good" for us has become more complex lately. Yes, studies of past meat intake, like the Harvard study I just mentioned, suggest a strong connection between red meat and disease. But when you think about how the red meat in those studies was raised, you have to wonder. The biggest problem with red meat may not turn out to be how much of it we eat, but what's in the feeding troughs of the animals we consume.

Traditionally, cows, pigs, sheep, and other farm animals ate grass. During the past few decades, however, livestock feed has been made up primarily of corn. In fact, many cattle are also fed waste products left over from the manufacturing of human food. These can include bakery waste, potato-processing remnant, untreated starch, pasta, and even candy. This type of feed fattens animals up fast because some of this processed feed is high in sugar and low in overall nutrients. I believe animals raised on highly processed feed produce meat that may contribute to some of the food-related chronic diseases plaguing Americans today.

When animals eat food like this, it sure makes sense to me that the people eating meat from these animals have higher rates of disease. I'm telling you not to load up on processed foods, baked goods, white pasta, and candy—so doesn't it make sense that the animals we eat shouldn't be consuming these foods either?

Wild meat—meat from game animals that eat natural food rather than processed grains—also seems to be much better for us than conventionally raised meat. Like grass-fed animals, wild animals such as deer, wild boar, and elk eat a huge range of whole, unprocessed foods.

I agree with scientists and food experts who say wild meat and the meat from grass-fed farm animals is much healthier for us than meat from animals raised on processed feed. It makes so much sense to me: unlike an animal that is force-fed unhealthy food, an animal that eats grass in a pasture consumes a huge range of nutrients from an array of greens.

A growing number of studies support grass feeding. For example, a 2011 study published in the *British Journal of Nutrition* found that subjects who ate grass-fed meat for just four weeks increased their blood levels of omega-3 fatty acids and decreased their levels of pro-inflammatory fatty acids. We don't usually think of meat as a source of omega-3 fatty acids, but when animals eat grass, they get more omega-3s in their diet.

And in 2009, researchers from Clemson University and the US Department of Agriculture looked closely at the effect of grass-fed beef on human health. Their study, published in the *Journal of Animal Science*, found that grass-fed beef is far healthier than conventionally raised beef. I don't ordinarily read studies in animal science journals, but believe me, that one caught my interest. The study found that compared with conventional beef, grass-fed beef is:

✚ Lower in total fat

✚ Higher in beta-carotene (an antioxidant found in vegetables)

✚ Higher in vitamin E

✚ Higher in the B vitamins thiamin and riboflavin

✚ Higher in the minerals calcium, magnesium, and potassium

✚ Higher in total omega-3s

✚ Higher in conjugated linoleic acid, a fatty acid that may fight disease

✚ Lower in the saturated fats linked with heart disease

But wait—before you run off and start eating red meat three times a day, I still feel that we have a lot to learn about red meat before we fully understand its impact on human health. We have studies suggesting that grass-fed meat is healthier—but we still don't know if those health benefits will result in lower disease rates.

Until we have a fuller picture of this evolving story, here's what I suggest: Limit your red meat intake to a few servings a week. When you do choose red meat, go for grass-fed or wild when possible. And limit your intake of processed meats.

Just so we're clear, processed meats are meats preserved by smoking, curing, salting, or with the addition of preservatives. I like the taste of bacon as much as anyone else, but I seldom eat it. I enjoy sausages, but you rarely find them on my plate as well. Same goes for ham, pastrami, salami, pepperoni, and hot dogs. They're tasty, but in my opinion, not worth the risk as a daily go-to option.

Why? The connection between colorectal cancer and eating processed meats is "startlingly strong," according to the American Institute of Cancer Research. When meat is processed, cured, smoked, or preserved, cancer-causing compounds can be formed.

Meat lovers smile at the thought of a perfectly grilled steak, a tasty piece of broiled chicken, or a yummy kabob of barbecued shrimp. I like those foods as much as the next guy or gal, but unfortunately, those cooking methods aren't the safest way to go.

When meat, poultry, and seafood are cooked and charred at high temperatures, as they are during grilling and broiling, the heat reacts with compounds in the meat to produce carcinogenic compounds known as heterocyclic amines (HCAs) and polycyclic aromatic hydrocarbons (PAHs). When consumed, HCAs and PAHs can damage DNA and contribute to the development of cancer of the colon and stomach.

This makes me uneasy about grilling and broiling meat. I think it's fine to grill occasionally, but I wouldn't recommend making grilling or broiling your everyday cooking method. Baking, poaching, stir-frying, and braising seem to be healthier choices.

Go ahead and grill fruits and vegetables, though—the compounds in meats that lead to carcinogen formation are not found in plant foods. You'd be amazed at how delicious grilled fruits and vegetables taste!

TIPS FOR HEALTHIER GRILLING

When you do opt to grill meat, poultry, and shellfish, follow these guidelines to help minimize the formation of carcinogens:

✚ Choose leaner cuts of meat, and trim off all visible fat, because dripping fat can cause fiery flare-ups that deposit carcinogenic compounds on food.

✚ Turn down the flames; fewer flames mean fewer carcinogens.

✚ Marinate meats for 30 minutes before grilling. Studies have shown that marinating meats before grilling can actually reduce the formation of carcinogens. The healthiest marinades contain nutrient-rich ingredients such as olive oil, vinegar, citrus juices, minced vegetables from the allium family (onions, chives, garlic, leeks), fresh herbs (rosemary, thyme, parsley, oregano, sage), and spices (turmeric, cumin, chili powder). Use paper towels to dry off excess marinade before cooking, because dripping marinade can cause flare-ups.

✚ Parboil meats before grilling—for example, poach chicken in boiling water until it's mostly cooked, and then finish it up on the grill.

✚ Flip meat often to reduce charring.

WRAP UP A PROTEIN-VEGGIE PACKET

Broiling or grilling meat in foil packets is one of my favorite cooking methods for poultry and fish. Not only does it protect your meat from forming HCAs and PAHs, but it is an easy, delicious way to make a nutritious protein and veggie meal without a lot of fuss or cleanup.

Here's how to do it: Place a piece of poultry or fish on the center part of a 12- by 18-inch piece of foil sprayed with cooking spray. Top with a serving of chopped fresh broccoli, cauliflower, red peppers, zucchini, or whatever vegetables you like. Drizzle with 1 teaspoon of oil (olive, sesame, peanut, or canola, depending on the taste you're going for) and sprinkle with fresh or dried herbs and/or spices to taste. Roll the top and ends of the foil together to seal the package well, but leave some room in the packet for air to circulate. Place on the grill or under the broiler and cook for 12 to 18 minutes, depending on the thickness of the poultry or fish. When it's ready to come off the heat, don't make the mistake of grabbing the hot-to-the-touch foil packet with your bare hands—a wide metal spatula works best for this—and be careful not to burn yourself on the steam emitting from the packet when you open it.

PROTEIN: A GREAT STRATEGY

There's no doubt about it: protein has the power to help you lose weight. And The Doctor's Diet is carefully designed to help you harness protein's power. No, you can't go crazy with protein, loading your plate with high-protein foods whenever you feel like it. But by using protein strategically—eating balanced amounts of it throughout your day in the most effective way possible—you can take full advantage of its ability to burn fat, fight hunger pangs, and rev up weight loss.

The story doesn't end with protein, though. The carbohydrates you eat (and don't eat) play a huge part in weight loss as well. That's why making smart choices about carbohydrates is my next Food Prescription.

FOOD PRESCRIPTION #3
CHOOSE SUPER-FILLING, FAT-BURNING CARBOHYDRATES

These days, when people peddling fad diets say the word "carbohydrate," they tend to get a sour look on their faces, as if they've just bitten into a very tart lemon. To them, carbohydrates should be avoided at just about all costs. It's all very black-and-white to them: Carbohydrates are bad. Staying away from them is good.

The only problem with this kind of anti-carbohydrate approach is that it reflects the old way of thinking that has been debunked by the scientific community.

Listen, when it comes to sugar, white flour, white bread, and many of the other simple sugars—I'll tell you more about them in a minute—I agree, you're better off without them. But there are plenty of good carbohydrates that you absolutely should be including in your meals. Foods like vegetables, fruits, legumes—even whole grains, which some fad diets wouldn't recommend in a million years.

The Doctor's Diet is different from a lot of the other eating plans out there because it includes a healthy assortment of complex carbohydrates. Not just vegetables, but beans and whole grains, such as a variety of whole-grain breads, cereals and pastas. That's because I believe—based on my reading of the medical literature and all of the study and analysis I've done in the area of dietary science—that cutting out a whole tribe of foods just because a few members of the family are troublemakers makes no sense whatsoever.

Yeah, there are a lot of unhealthy carbohydrates. But there are some pretty great ones, too. I just don't believe that avoiding all carbohydrates is the way to go for enjoying long-term health, not to mention the enjoyment of eating. And I think they should be a part of your diet, so I give them an important role in The Doctor's Diet.

One of the arguments made by the anti-carbohydrate camp is that cutting out carbs speeds up weight loss. There's some truth to that. But like so many things in life, it's not as simple as it sounds. Yes, cutting out *simple* carbs helps rev up weight loss. But it's not necessary to push *complex* carbs off your plate. You can lose weight and burn fat while still enjoying the many health benefits of fruits, vegetables, legumes, and whole grains. You just have to make smart choices about which carbs you eat and how they balance out with the protein and fat in your diet.

Follow The Doctor's Diet and your meals will contain the best combination of high-fiber carbohydrates, fat-burning protein, and appetite-satisfying fat.

SHOULD YOU GO GLUTEN-FREE?

Unless you have celiac disease (a condition in which the gluten in wheat, rye, and barley actually causes physical damage to your intestines) or an intolerance to gluten (which can cause bloating, nausea, or other symptoms), there's no reason to cut out gluten-containing grains from your diet.

Eating gluten-free is a fad right now, with lots of so-called nutrition experts telling people that everyone should avoid it. But despite what you may have heard, there's simply no evidence to suggest that a wholesale banishment of gluten from your diet is a good idea.

In fact, eating gluten-free breads, cereals, and other grain-based foods instead of whole-wheat versions is likely to lower the quality of your diet rather than raise it. Many gluten-free products are made with rice flour, potato flour, tapioca, and other simple carbohydrates rather than whole grains. Often, manufacturers use excess sugar and fat to cover up the less-than-appetizing tastes of the gluten-free ingredients, which lowers their nutritional value even more.

And don't get me started on rice milk, which is basically made from boiled white rice and sugar—nothing good in there.

I find it ironic that people who go gluten-free without really thinking it through often end up worsening their diets rather than improving them, because they are unknowingly taking healthy whole grains out of their diet and replacing them with simple carbs.

If your doctor has advised you to follow a gluten-free diet, by all means, follow that advice. I've included plenty of gluten-free options in The Doctor's Diet, because millions of Americans do better without having gluten in their system. But remember, eating gluten-free isn't an excuse to fill up on sugary carbohydrates, white breads, white rice, and lots of refined grain products. There are plenty of gluten-free whole grains available, including quinoa, gluten-free oats, millet, and amaranth. (Oats contain no gluten, but they are often stored and shipped with other grains and can become contaminated with gluten. To avoid cross-contamination, choose oats with "gluten-free" on the label.)

Q: WHAT IS FOOD INTOLERANCE, AND HOW DO I KNOW IF I CAN'T TOLERATE SPECIFIC TYPES OF FOODS?

A: People with food intolerances notice various kinds of symptoms after eating a certain food or foods. They may have gastrointestinal reactions (gas, bloating, nausea, vomiting, diarrhea, cramps, stomach pain, heartburn) or a change in how they feel overall—irritable, tired, or just "off." To determine whether you have an intolerance to a food, don't eat it for a while; then introduce it back into your diet and notice how it makes you feel. If symptoms occur, you may want to avoid eating it. Food intolerances are different from food allergies, which can be life threatening. Food allergies can cause some of the same symptoms as food intolerance, but allergic reactions tend to occur soon after the food has been eaten. An allergic reaction may include difficulty breathing or swallowing, skin rash or hives, rapidly beating heart, swelling of the eyes and throat, and other scary reactions. If this happens, go to the hospital or call 911.

THE SIMPLE TRUTH ABOUT CARBS

Your body uses the carbohydrates in food for energy. It breaks carbohydrates down into glucose, which is the fuel your cells need to function.

There are two kinds of carbohydrates: complex and simple. In a nutshell, you're best off cutting back on simple carbohydrates and focusing on complex carbohydrates. Here's why:

COMPLEX CARBOHYDRATES

Complex carbohydrates are, as their name implies, complex. They provide a more gradual energy source than simple carbohydrates and are more likely to come from whole, natural foods that have not been processed and stripped of their God-given, nutrient-rich components. Foods that contain healthy amounts of complex carbohydrates include vegetables, legumes, and whole grains.

Complex carbohydrates can boost your health by providing vitamins, minerals, and a range of phytonutrients, as well as fiber.

Your body does convert the complex carbohydrates in food into glucose for fuel, but it takes longer than it does for simple carbs. As a result, when you eat foods with complex carbohydrates, glucose enters your bloodstream slowly and gradually, rather than with a sudden, near-instantaneous spike.

SIMPLE CARBOHYDRATES

Simple carbohydrates are exactly what their name suggests: simple. Often they are refined, which means their complexity has been stripped away by food manufacturers and processing. The most famous example of a simple carbohydrate is table sugar, but simple carbohydrates are also found in white bread, white rice, white pasta, cakes, cookies, pastries, sugar-sweetened soft drinks, and candy. Simple carbohydrates from processed foods and sugar make weight gain easier and weight loss more difficult. They also raise the risk of heart disease and diabetes.

When you eat simple carbohydrates, your body converts them to glucose very quickly. That glucose gets dumped into your bloodstream rapidly, causing a quick rise in blood sugar and insulin.

Simple carbohydrates also include natural sugars found in plant foods (fruits and, in small amounts, some vegetables) and dairy products. Although these carbohydrates are simple, they are in a different category than simple sugars such as white sugar, brown sugar, corn syrup, and others that are added to foods. That's because they contain other components (vitamins, proteins and minerals in dairy, and an abundance of phytochemicals and fiber in fruit) that make them way more valuable than sugary, processed foods.

Fiber is a type of carbohydrate that can't be digested by your body. It passes through your body without being broken down into glucose.

There are two kinds of fiber: soluble and insoluble. Plant foods can have one or both kinds of fiber, and both are important for your health. Soluble fiber is found in oatmeal, oat bran, nuts, seeds, most fruits, and legumes. Insoluble fiber comes from whole-wheat bread, barley, brown rice, bulgur, whole-grain cereals, wheat bran, seeds, and most fruits and vegetables.

Fiber is crucial for a few reasons. For one, it actually helps get rid of fat in your digestive system—think of it as a scrub brush that travels through your intestines clearing away some of the excess fat and cholesterol that's floating around. It also helps move things along as they should in your intestines, which helps prevent constipation and promotes good bowel health. Eating foods that are high in fiber helps you feel full longer, keeping hunger pangs at bay and helping you lose weight and keep it off. And because fiber slows down the digestion of carbohydrates, it helps keep blood sugar stable.

Studies show that people who eat a high-fiber diet are less likely to develop type 2 diabetes than those who don't. High-fiber foods also seem to lower the risk of heart disease.

Q: HOW MUCH FIBER SHOULD I GET EACH DAY?

A: The Institute of Medicine guidelines for dietary fiber are:

✚ Men 50 and younger - 38g/day

✚ Men 51 and older - 30g/day

✚ Women 50 and younger - 25g/day

✚ Women 51 and older - 21g/day

FIBER IN FOODS

FIBER SOURCE	GRAMS OF FIBER
1 medium apple, with peel	3
1 medium banana	3
1 cup blueberries	4
½ medium grapefruit	4
1 cup melon	1
1 medium pear, with peel	4-5
1 cup raspberries or blackberries	8
1 cup strawberries	3
½ cup most cooked vegetables (asparagus, green beans, broccoli, cauliflower, eggplant, greens, squash, tomato)	1-3
½ cup cooked beans (black, kidney, pinto, etc.)	5-8
1 medium sweet potato	3
1 slice whole-grain bread	2-3
½ cup bran and other very high-fiber cereals	10-14
½ cup oatmeal	2
1 ounce nuts or 2 tablespoons nut butter	2-4
½ cup cooked barley	3
½ cup brown rice	2
2 tablespoons toasted wheat germ	3

Q: SHOULD I AVOID WHITE POTATOES BECAUSE OF THEIR HIGH STARCH CONTENT?

A: You can have them occasionally, because they do contain nutrients (they are a great source of potassium). But in general, white potatoes are similar to white bread, white rice, and other "white" foods that are converted to glucose very quickly and raise blood sugar. If you're hankering for potatoes, have a small amount, choose baked rather than fried (often fried potatoes are cooked with trans fats), and make sure to pair them with foods that contain protein, fiber, and healthy fats, which will help offset their effect on your blood sugar. Or choose colorful potatoes (purple, for example), whose bright colors deliver a dose of antioxidants.

WHOLE GRAINS

Whole grains are grains that have not had their fibrous or nutritious parts removed. Some kinds of whole grains include:

- Barley
- Brown rice
- Buckwheat
- Bulgur
- Corn
- Millet
- Oats/oatmeal

- Popcorn (choose air-popped without additives)
- Quinoa
- Rye
- Triticale
- Whole wheat
- Wild rice

PUT CARBS TO WORK FOR YOU

So many people have said so many bad things about carbs lately, but as you can see, there's no reason to give them up. In fact, you can make carbohydrates work for you, giving them a major position on your weight-loss team. The trick is to eat the right kinds of carbs—and now you know which ones will do the most heavy lifting for you.

As I said earlier, The Doctor's Diet is different from many of the other eating plans out there because it builds in a healthy assortment of complex and healthy carbohydrates including fruits, whole grains, beans, and fresh vegetables.

I'll tell you more about this, but before I do, we've got to pay some attention to the big, white elephant in the room: sugar. Don't worry, I'll be as sweet about it as I can.

The most notorious simple carbohydrate—and one of the major causes of excess weight and poor health—is sitting in a bowl in your kitchen. It's pure and white, sparkly and sweet—but don't let its innocent appearance fool you. No matter how benign it may look, sugar is just plain bad for you, and cutting it out of your diet—if not completely, then mostly—will not only help you lose weight and cut your risk of disease, but it will probably make you feel a whole lot better, too.

Most of us eat way too much sugar. The American Heart Association recommends limiting added sugar to no more than 100 calories a day for women and 150 calories a day for men. But we Americans consume, on average, 355 calories from sugar each day—that's about 22 teaspoons of sugar daily. Over the course of a year, that's enough calories to pack on 37 extra pounds!

But we're not sitting around munching on sugar cubes or spooning the white stuff into our mouths from our sugar bowls—rather, we're consuming it in the food we eat and the beverages we drink. Sugar is found in the expected places, such as cookies, candy, cakes, muffins, ice cream, sugary cereals, and pastries. And it's in foods we don't necessarily think of as being very sugary, such as breads, pastas and many sauces and dressings. And of course, it's in soft drinks—soda, sweetened iced tea, sports drinks, fruit punches, lemonade, sugary coffee drinks, and other kinds of "liquid candy."

Our bodies are biologically programmed to seek out the taste of sweetness. Back when our cavemen ancestors were roaming the forests, seashores, and prairies, sweetness equaled safety—in general, if something tasted sweet, it was unlikely to be poisonous. A sugary taste was linked with good health and long life, which is a bitter irony when you consider how many modern lives are shortened because of our desire for sugar.

Today we've still got that physiological urge to eat sweets. But now we live in a world in which sugar is everywhere. We can't just go by what our bodies want. We've got to change the way we think about sugar, root it out of our diets, and break what is, for many of us, an addiction.

Nutrition experts disagree over whether the constant, overwhelming craving for sugar that so many of us have is an addiction—meaning a true physiological dependence—or just a bad habit. My view is that it's an addiction, an actual physical craving, and that a sizeable number of people truly are addicted to sugar.

When an overweight person with life-threatening heart disease and type 2 diabetes hides candy bars around the house, eats them when nobody's looking, and then weeps with self-hatred afterward, I call that an addiction.

Here's my thinking. When you're addicted to something, you have trouble controlling your use of it. You continue to use it, take it, or consume it despite realizing that it's harmful to your health. Even when you try to give it up, you may find that you can't. Powerful cravings leave you thinking of it constantly, but consuming it gives you only fleeting satisfaction.

When we think of addictions, substances like alcohol, nicotine, and recreational drugs come to mind, as do gambling and sex addiction. But for some people, sugar can be just as addictive.

Eating sugar causes your brain to release serotonin and dopamine, brain chemicals that make you feel good. These same neurochemicals are produced when you fall in love, have sex, or experience any kind of pleasure. And, not surprisingly, they are released in the brains of people who use drugs such as cocaine and heroin.

Eating high-sugar food actually stimulates an entire region of the brain that's known as the reward center. Not all foods do this—in fact, an impressive 2013 study published in the *American Journal of Clinical Nutrition* found that foods that are high on the glycemic index (in other words, foods that are high in sugar) stimulate the brain's reward and craving regions significantly more than foods that are low in sugar.

It's a simple equation. You eat sugar, you feel good, your brain fires off "pleasure" signals, you eat more sugar—and the cycle goes on and on.

Blood sugar plays a part as well. Again, the equation is simple: you eat sugar, your blood sugar skyrockets, your blood sugar plummets, your brain turns on a low blood sugar alert, and before you know it you're craving sugar again.

That's what happened to me when I was a kid. I grew up drinking tons of sugar, and I truly believe I was addicted to it because I felt like I couldn't live without it. What a relief it was for me to break that addiction and not have to feel so beholden to all those bottles of soda.

The problem with sugar is that it's ubiquitous—it's all around us. Alcoholics who get off booze can avoid bars, nightclubs, and parties where it's served, and recovering drug addicts don't have to worry that there's cocaine in their spaghetti sauce! Not so with sugar. It's in the vast majority of processed foods—as well as just about every kitchen, restaurant, coffee shop, and convenience store—so it's nearly impossible to avoid it completely.

You *can* break your addiction to sugar. Once you decide that you really do want to end your psychological dependence on this life-threatening food, you can end sugar's control on your body and your taste buds. Then, once you're free of the constant desire for sweetness, you'll find it much easier to enjoy the naturally delicious taste of whole foods that are better for you and that help you burn excess fat.

I GREW UP DRINKING TONS OF SUGAR, AND I TRULY BELIEVE I WAS ADDICTED TO IT BECAUSE I FELT LIKE I COULDN'T LIVE WITHOUT IT. WHAT A RELIEF IT WAS FOR ME TO BREAK THAT ADDICTION AND NOT HAVE TO FEEL SO BEHOLDEN TO ALL THOSE BOTTLES OF SODA.

BREAKING YOUR SUGAR ADDICTION

Ending your psychological reliance on sugar isn't easy, but it's absolutely doable. I've created a five-step process that will help you end your sugar addiction.

STEP 1: FIGURE OUT WHETHER YOU'RE ADDICTED.

I'm not sure if it's because of genetics or just the way we're raised, but it definitely seems that some people are more likely to become addicted to sugar than others. How do you rate? Are you someone who wakes up in a sweat after dreaming of chocolate cream pie? Are you immune to sugar—can you easily say "no thanks" to candy, cookies, and desserts? Or are you, like most people, somewhere in the middle? Take this quiz to find out where you stand. Circle the answer that most closely fits each question.

1. Do you eat sweets even when you're not hungry?

Very frequently   Somewhat frequently   Occasionally   Never

2. Do you go overboard on sweets, eating three or more servings of cake, cookies, candy, ice cream, or other sweets at one time?

Very frequently   Somewhat frequently   Occasionally   Never

3. When you're eating something sweet, do you continue to consume it even after you start feeling full?

Very frequently   Somewhat frequently   Occasionally   Never

4. Do you become defensive when friends and family comment about your intake of cookies, candy, cake, and other sweets?

Very frequently   Somewhat frequently   Occasionally   Never

5. Do you lie to others about your intake of sugary foods? For example, if you eat a bunch of cookies and another family member is wondering why the cookie box is empty, do you fib to cover up the fact that you ate them?

Very frequently   Somewhat frequently   Occasionally   Never

6. Do you experience withdrawal-type symptoms (irritability, moodiness, depression, anxiety, etc.) when you try to give up sweets?

Very frequently   Somewhat frequently   Occasionally   Never

7. Do you have candy and other sweets stashed around the house where others can't find them, and do you eat them when nobody is watching?

Very frequently   Somewhat frequently   Occasionally   Never

8. Do you feel ashamed, guilty, or angry at yourself when you eat/overeat sugary foods?

Very frequently   Somewhat frequently   Occasionally   Never

9. Do you find yourself thinking about sweets throughout the day and night, counting the minutes until it's "time" to eat them?

Very frequently   Somewhat frequently   Occasionally   Never

10. Do you automatically reach for something sweet after finishing a meal?

Very frequently   Somewhat frequently   Occasionally   Never

11. Do you feel panicked or desperate when you don't have something sweet in the house for dessert?

Very frequently   Somewhat frequently   Occasionally   Never

12. Do you *think* you may be addicted to sugar and sweets?

Very frequently   Somewhat frequently   Occasionally   Never

Scoring: Give yourself the following points for each answer you circled, then use the chart that follows to determine the likelihood that you're addicted to sugar:

Very frequently: 3 points

Occasionally: 1 point

Somewhat frequently: 2 points

Never: 0 points

SCORE	WHAT IT MEANS
0-8	You're one of the lucky ones—you can typically pass up sweets easily and are probably not addicted.
9-16	You struggle with sweet eating. Although you are sometimes in control, at other times you are pulled into addictive behavior by your desire for sugar.
17-24	Sugar is definitely a problem for you. Although you may not be experiencing full-fledged addiction, your mind and body rely heavily on sugar.
25-36	You are most likely addicted to sugar.

STEP 2: IDENTIFY THE ADDED SUGAR IN YOUR DIET.

Even if you're not loading up on cake and pie or drinking can after can of soda, you're probably taking in much more sugar than you realize. That's because sugar is added to so many foods—even the ones we don't think of as being sweet, such as spaghetti sauce, frozen dinners, and salad dressings. Sugar boosts flavor, tones down bitterness, and balances the sharpness of high-acid foods such as tomatoes and vinegar. It also helps preserve foods, which is one of the reasons it's in so many processed products.

To find the hidden (and not-so-hidden) sugar in the foods you eat, start reading labels. The Nutrition Facts section of the label gives you total grams of sugar, but that includes natural sugars as well as added sugars. For example, according to the food label, a cup of skim milk has 12 grams of sugar. But that all comes from lactose, a natural sugar in milk. Although some people think you need to cut out lactose and other natural sugars in order to break your addiction to sugar, I don't agree.

So when you're looking at food labels, consider the total amount of sugar grams, but more importantly, look at the food's ingredients. If sugar is one of the food's first ingredients, consider avoiding it.

But you have to be on your toes. When sugar is added to a food, the word "sugar" may not even appear on its label. That's because on food labels, sugar often hides behind a range of different names. When you see these words on labels, sugar alarm bells should go off in your head:

- agave nectar
- barley malt
- beet sugar
- brown rice syrup
- brown sugar
- cane juice
- cane sugar
- cane syrup
- corn sugar
- corn sweeteners
- corn syrup
- date sugar
- dextran
- dextrose
- evaporated cane juice
- fructose
- fruit juice concentrate
- fruit nectars
- glucose
- glucose solids
- high-fructose corn syrup
- honey
- invert sugar
- lactose
- malt syrup
- maltose
- maple syrup
- molasses
- rice syrup
- sorghum syrup
- sucrose syrup
- turbinado sugar

STEP 3: MAKE THE DECISION TO CUT OUT SUGAR.

You may be thinking, "But Dr. Travis, I've already made the decision to stop eating sugar—in fact, I've made it about a million times!" That's OK. I know it's hard. But I'm talking about really making a choice here, committing to it and telling yourself you're really going to follow through. You might even want to write yourself a letter or make a contract with yourself—doing something formal like that can move the decision from something you kind of want to do to something you absolutely are deciding to do.

There are two ways to cut excess sugar from your diet: gradually and cold turkey. Opinions differ on which is the better way to go, but here's where I stand: do whatever works for you. And it's OK if you don't know which path to take—you can try both approaches and see how you fare. The goal is to get all that extra sugar out of your diet, and as long as you reach that goal, I don't really care how you do it.

Some people feel great waking up one day and saying, "That's it, no more extra sugar!" and they're all ready to jump on the bandwagon for good. If this is how you want to approach it, go for it.

But an all-at-once approach isn't for everyone. If you're consuming a large amount of sugar—say you're drinking multiple cans of soda or sweetened iced tea every day—going cold turkey may not work for you, especially if you're also taking in a lot of caffeine. Doing so could lead to headaches, irritability, and other symptoms. For heavy-duty sugar users, cutting back on sugar over a series of days (or even weeks) may work better for you.

Go with your gut, and use whatever method will bring you the most success.

STEP 4: CHOOSE LOW-SUGAR ALTERNATIVES.

Once you uncover the added sugar in your diet, choose naturally low-sugar foods that contain little or no added sugar. For example, if your breakfast cereal has lots of sugar, choose a different type, but not one with artificial sweetener (which I will discuss more next). If your favorite tomato sauce is high in sugar, pick a different brand—or better yet, make your own out of fresh or canned tomatoes. Same with your salad dressing—instead of something with high-fructose corn syrup or other sweeteners, just splash your salad with olive oil and balsamic vinegar mixed with chopped fresh herbs.

If you usually drink soda, sweetened iced tea, or other sugary beverages, switch to plain water, unsweetened tea, or unsweetened seltzer with a dash of fruit juice or real fruit.

Look, I'm not going to tell you that you can't *ever* have sugar. But I do think you should cut as much added sugar out of your diet as possible. Our bodies are simply not designed to process all the sugar in the typical American diet. When you look at the rising rates of most chronic diseases, they correspond with a similar increase of sugar intake among Americans.

Do your best to cut added sugars out of your diet. If you do need a little bit of sweetness in your coffee or oatmeal, choose honey, molasses or maple syrup, which contain antioxidants. That way, at least you'll get a little something good, too.

Notice I'm not suggesting you replace sugars with artificial sweeteners. I have real concerns about artificial sweeteners—the fat-free craze of the 1990s coincided with a massive uptick in their use, and studies suggest an association between artificial sweeteners and obesity and type 2 diabetes. Artificial sweeteners are just another part of our fascination with overly sweet foods.

You'd think that since they have few or no calories, artificial sweeteners would help with weight loss. But some studies suggest that's simply not the case. For example, guzzling diet soda is actually associated with an elevated risk of obesity and type 2 diabetes. This is the conclusion of a number of studies, including an analytic review of research published in July 2013 in the journal *Trends in Endocrinology*. Researchers think artificial sweeteners trick your body into thinking it is consuming real sugar, which causes your body to release insulin and store belly fat. On top of that, artificial sweeteners may also contribute to carbohydrate cravings.

Do I think it's going to kill you if you consume artificial sweeteners occasionally? No—but I firmly believe they play a part in setting your taste buds up to expect highly sweetened foods all the time and to crave sweets and simple carbohydrates.

I also believe that giving up artificial sweeteners helps reset your palate so it's back to normal, able to appreciate the natural tastes of whole foods rather than always demanding hyper-sweet, sugar-laden foods.

I've seen this happen myself: anytime I've had diet soda and then fruit, I've noticed that the fruit tastes unusually bland. Even after just one diet soda, I can feel my taste buds getting reset in the *wrong* direction. This is why now and going forward, I personally avoid all artificial sweeteners.

One of my goals in The Doctor's Diet is to help you reset your palate so you can go back to enjoying the natural, more subtle sweetness of whole foods such as fruits. It's something I had to learn, and I know you can too.

ABOUT 80 PERCENT OF ALL PACKAGED FOODS IN THE UNITED STATES CONTAIN ADDED SUGARS.

Once you stop eating sweets, you'll start having cravings. That's OK—it's normal and it's part of the process. The cravings may be strong at first, but believe me, they'll start to weaken after the first couple of days, and before you know it, they'll disappear. Once your body recognizes that you're not going to give in to sugar cravings, they begin to lose their power over you.

In the meantime, make a list of activities you can do to distract yourself when cravings hit. If you truly are hungry, eat a healthy, high-protein snack. If you're thirsty, drink a big glass of water. If you're simply bored or just craving something sweet, take your mind off it. Call a friend, go for a walk, play with your dog, jump on your bicycle, take a bubble bath, put on some music and dance around the living room, read a trashy novel—do whatever it takes to occupy your mind until the craving passes, because it will pass. And when it does, you'll feel great about yourself for getting through it without giving in.

If you make mistakes, forgive yourself and move on. Don't berate yourself or wallow in self-blame. Just stop yourself, put down the cookie, recommit to your goal, and start fresh.

It really is amazing how quickly you start to lose your cravings and your taste for sugar. The truth is that the more sugar you eat, the more you want—but the opposite is true as well, and the *less* sugar you eat, the *less* you want! Before you know it, the foods you used to love because of their sweetness will taste overly sweet. Your taste buds adjust, your brain adjusts, and you move on to a new kind of sweetness as you savor a healthier life and a leaner body.

ADDED VS. NATURAL

Sugar is a type of carbohydrate that your body uses for energy. When it's found naturally in foods such as fruits, dairy foods, grains, and some vegetables, it's referred to as "natural sugar." When it's added to foods, it's referred to as "added sugar." Makes sense, right?

Some people think that natural sugar and added sugar are equally bad for you. But I don't agree. The sugar that occurs naturally in fruits and other foods is not what worries me. America doesn't have an obesity epidemic because people are eating too many apples and oranges. It's because they're drinking too much soda, eating too many sweets, and consuming vast amounts of sugar in processed foods.

HERE'S WHY IT'S CALLED "LIQUID CANDY." A 12-OUNCE CAN OF SUGAR-SWEETENED COLA CONTAINS 39 GRAMS (NINE TEASPOONS) OF SUGAR. PEOPLE WHO HAVE SUGARY DRINKS DAILY—ONE TO TWO CANS A DAY OR MORE—HAVE A 26 PERCENT GREATER RISK OF DEVELOPING TYPE 2 DIABETES THAN DO PEOPLE WHO RARELY CONSUME SUGARY DRINKS.

Go ahead and enjoy fruit, but be very careful when it comes to processed foods with a lot of added sugar. Here's why:

✚ **Added sugar contributes to weight gain.** People who eat added sugar are more likely to become overweight or obese. The more sugar they eat, the more they gain.

✚ **Added sugar increases your risk of developing type 2 diabetes.** Eating too much sugar can interfere with your body's ability to process insulin. This can lead to insulin resistance and type 2 diabetes.

✚ **Added sugar prevents your brain from hearing the "I'm full" signal.** Large sugar intake leads to the production of excess insulin, which can prevent leptin, the appetite-control hormone, from signaling to our brains that we should stop eating.

✚ **Added sugar calories are empty calories.** There's no nutritional value in them whatsoever, and they paradoxically can make you feel less full.

✚ **Added sugar displaces nutritious foods.** The more sugar you eat, the less room there is in your diet for healthy foods such as vegetables, fruits, legumes, nuts, and whole grains.

✦ **Added sugar has dangerous friends.** Many processed foods that contain large amounts of added sugar also have trans fats (more on this later), artificial flavors and colors, and other unhealthy ingredients that contribute to poor health.

✦ **Added sugar raises heart disease risk.** Quite simply, excess added sugar turns to fat in our bodies. That's why too much sugar increases belly fat and raises triglycerides, and LDL ("bad") cholesterol, which amps up your chances of heart disease.

SUGAR BY THE NUMBERS

1 teaspoon of table sugar = 4.2 grams sugar = 16 calories

GETTING IN CONTROL

It's no surprise that so many of us are addicted to sugar. Eating sugar stimulates your brain's reward center and triggers the release of feel-good brain chemicals. And because sugar is everywhere, it can be difficult to break its grip on you.

Facing down a sugar addiction is definitely a challenge—but it's something you can do. Once you understand the hold that sugar has on you, and once you decide to start taking steps to free yourself from sugar's stranglehold on your diet, you really can take charge. By following the steps I've outlined here, you can free yourself from sugar's grasp and open yourself up to the naturally delicious flavors of healthy foods.

No, it won't be easy. But look back at your life and count up all the difficult challenges you've confronted, all the victories you've achieved. You've done harder things than breaking up with sugar. And you're stronger than you realize! Do this now and you'll achieve one of the sweetest wins of your life!

If you've tried losing weight before, you've probably gone down the low-fat fad road. You've tried all those rubbery fat-free cheeses, the cardboard-like fat-free cookies, the bizarrely tasteless fat-free chips, the thin, flavorless fat-free ice creams. You've been there, and I'm guessing you're not particularly interested in going there again.

Well, you can relax. One of the great things about The Doctor's Diet is that it's not a super low-fat diet. Sure, we keep an eye on the amount of fat you're eating because fat has a fair amount of calories, and we've got to keep calories in check in order to bring down weight. But there's no reason in the world to cut all fat out of your diet. In fact, eliminating fat is actually a really bad idea.

I'm not saying you can lose weight by eating unlimited amounts of full-fat cheese and snack foods—definitely not. But you can—and should—eat adequate amounts of healthy fats in order to bring down your weight as well as your risk of disease.

FAT FACTS

When it comes to dietary fat, there are three really important things you need to know right off the bat.

1. FAT IS NOT THE ENEMY!

For years we were told that dietary fat was just about the worst thing you could eat. Scientists said it. Fad diet opportunists said it. Even the most well-meaning doctors said it. We all thought it was true, and we advised people to cut out as much fat as possible from their diets. But when people ditched all the fat in their diets, researchers were amazed to see that health problems actually got worse rather than better. Super low-fat diets didn't eliminate heart disease or cause people to thin down to healthy weights overnight. More careful research told us what we now know: although some kinds of fat are not healthy, and although we do have to limit our overall fat intake because of the calories it contains, there is actually no reason at all to cut every bit of fat from our diets. In fact, some kinds of dietary fat are incredibly good for us, and by leaving them off our plates, we're missing out on some amazing nutrients.

2. LOW-FAT AND FAT-FREE FOOD SUBSTITUTES CAN ACTUALLY BE **WORSE** FOR YOU THAN THE FULL-FAT FOODS THEY REPLACE.

That's right—replacing full-fat foods with highly processed, commercially manufactured low-fat or fat-free alternatives—fat-free cookies, chips, cakes, some kinds of cheeses, and so on—actually can cause more harm than good. When people eat a low-fat diet, they typically cut out the good fats as well as the bad fats. And they eat way more sugar, simple carbs, and artificial fillers.

3. EATING FAT DOES NOT MAKE YOU FAT.

In fact, including a healthy amount of fat in your meals can actually satiate your hunger and help you lose weight. If you've ever suffered through the agony of a salad tossed with fat-free dressing, I can't wait to tell you about the studies that show that olive oil–based salad dressing can be a better weight-loss tool than the fat-free sludge that's sold in the name of good health.

It's time to stop fearing fat and start being smart about it. As long as you know what kind of fat to eat, how much fat to eat, and how to include it in your diet in the healthiest way—which is what I do in The Doctor's Diet—you no longer have to think of fat as your enemy. Instead, consider it an ally in your quest for weight loss and good health.

WHEN PEOPLE EAT A LOW-FAT DIET, THEY TYPICALLY CUT OUT THE GOOD FATS AS WELL AS THE BAD FATS. AND THEY EAT WAY MORE SUGAR, SIMPLE CARBS, AND ARTIFICIAL FILLERS.

THE SKINNY ON FATS

All fat is not created equal. Some are good for you, some aren't. So let's start with a quick look at the various kinds of dietary fats.

SATURATED FAT

For a long time, scientists believed saturated fat—the kind found in meat, full-fat cheese, butter, cow's milk, cream, ice cream, and palm and coconut oils—was a major cause of heart disease. But that belief has undergone a seismic shift recently, as researchers have learned more about saturated fat. As it turns out, the connection between saturated fat and heart disease is more complex than we previously thought.

Here's the current thinking. Saturated fat raises LDL cholesterol, which is bad for your heart. But it also seems to raise HDL cholesterol and lower triglycerides, which is good for your heart.

In effect, current research shows that saturated fat can have both a positive and negative impact on heart health. Recent population studies (i.e., studies of large numbers of people over long periods of time) back this up: they are finding that there is no significant evidence that saturated fat intake is associated with an increased risk of heart disease. It doesn't seem to raise risk, and it also doesn't seem to lower risk.

Of course, we saw hints of this awhile back when the French paradox first came to light. The French paradox is the discovery that the French have lower heart disease rates than their high-saturated-fat diet would suggest, leading researchers to wonder if saturated fat really is a cause of heart disease.

Separately, we also know that monounsaturated fat (found in fish, nuts, olive oil, avocado, and the like) is good for your heart. Studies of people who include ample unsaturated fats in their diet find that they lower heart disease risk.

So where does that leave us—should we go ahead and eat saturated fat, or stay away from it?

The answer is, it depends on what you're comparing it to. I don't mean to be coy here, but this really is a complicated question. Here's what it comes down to: When people replace saturated fat with healthier unsaturated fats, it benefits their heart health. But if they replace them with simple carbohydrates, trans fats, and other unhealthful foods, it harms their heart health.

As it appears now, saturated fat can be both good and bad—in other words, neutral. But unsaturated fat is good. And trans fat is bad. So whether saturated fat is a better choice really comes down to what you're comparing it to.

Think of it this way. You're looking at a dinner menu with three choices, each with an equal number of calories: fried chicken that's breaded and cooked in shortening that contains trans fat, sirloin steak, and baked salmon. Which should you order?

The salmon is the best choice, because it's loaded with heart-healthy omega-3 fatty acids that help your heart. The sirloin steak, which contains saturated fat, may be heart-health neutral. And if it's from a grass-fed cow, that's even better. But the fried chicken is flat-out bad for your heart.

So compared to the fried chicken, the grass-fed sirloin is a better choice. But compared to the sirloin, the salmon is a better choice.

My advice? Order the salmon most of the time. Have a steak occasionally. Avoid fried chicken pretty much all the time. In other words, keep saturated fat to a minimum, but it's OK to enjoy it occasionally. Think of red meat, butter, full-fat dairy foods, and other high-saturated fat foods as things you eat occasionally in smaller amounts.

It boils down to making sensible choices. I'd rather you choose natural foods with some saturated fat over unnatural foods filled with simple carbs and trans fats. Have a little bit of real ice cream instead of a big bowl of the fake stuff. Nibble on a small square of real cheddar cheese rather than a giant slice of the fat-free junk that tastes like plastic. Sauté your broccoli in a bit of butter rather than a pool of margarine. You get the idea.

But don't close the book on saturated fat yet. I think we're going to be hearing more about this topic in the near future as researchers study it more closely, so stay tuned as we learn more.

> **I'D RATHER YOU CHOOSE NATURAL FOODS WITH SOME SATURATED FAT OVER UNNATURAL FOODS FILLED WITH SIMPLE CARBS AND TRANS FATS.**

TRANS FAT

I'm not big on using the word "bad" when it comes to food, because I don't like taking such an absolute black-and-white viewpoint. But I make an exception for trans fat, because it really is bad. Trans fat, which is also known as trans fatty acids, is found naturally in small amounts in meat and dairy products—but I'm not really concerned about that. The trans fat that I really don't like is the stuff created in factories by food manufacturers. It's not just bad; it's terrible for you.

Most of the trans fat in the American diet come from artificially processed sources—foods that contain partially hydrogenated oil, which is formed by a manufacturing process called hydrogenation, in which hydrogen is added to liquid oil in order to turn it into a solid fat.

Food companies use hydrogenated trans fat for a variety of reasons. Not only is it cheaper than other kinds of fats, but it also helps prevent spoilage, which allows foods to stay fresh longer. It also gives foods an appealing texture, making pie crusts flakier, French fries crispier, and crackers crunchier. Hydrogenated fat is also used in some kinds of margarines, cake frostings, and other foods with a creamy texture.

It also greatly ups your heart attack risk because it raises LDL ("bad") cholesterol, raises triglyceride levels (which are better off being lower), and lowers HDL ("good") cholesterol. And that's a trifecta *none* of us wants!

Even small amounts seem to be detrimental to heart health. A major study found that heart disease risk went up by 50 percent in women who ate just four teaspoons a day of stick margarine made with trans fat. Trans fat contributes to thousands of heart attacks and heart disease deaths each year in the United States.

Eating trans fat also seems to mess with your blood sugar and insulin response and can turn up the heat on systemic inflammation—more reason to stay away from it, since systemic inflammation plays a part in a range of chronic diseases, from heart disease to cancer.

As we've become more aware of the danger of trans fats, their use has gone down, thank goodness. Some local governments now restrict their use, and as a result, many manufacturers have reformulated their products to be trans fat–free. But trans fats can still be found in many foods, including some kinds of microwave popcorn, frozen pizzas, commercially produced baked goods (cake, cookies, pies), some margarines and spreads, and some kinds of coffee creamers.

Dietary guidelines from the Institute of Medicine recommend eliminating as much trans fat from your diet as possible. That's a recommendation I agree with wholeheartedly—I suggest aiming for zero trans fat (except for the small amounts found in meat and dairy foods).

You can cut out trans fat by choosing whole, natural foods instead of processed, commercially manufactured foods. Use olive oil—or even a small amount of butter—instead of margarine, or choose trans fat–free olive oil margarines instead.

Keep in mind that trans fats can hide in foods. Labeling rules allow foods with less than 0.5 grams of trans fat per serving to be labeled "trans fat free" even if they contain small amounts of trans fats. Crazy, I know. But that's what we've got. So in order to make sure you're staying away from trans fats, ignore the marketing claims on the front of food packaging and instead look at ingredient lists on the back. If anywhere on the ingredient list says "partially hydrogenated oil" or "shortening," then I leave it on the store shelf. You should, too.

UNSATURATED FAT

Now let's look at the good kind of fat: the unsaturated kind. Unsaturated fats are the healthy fats, the ones that play a major role in a healthy diet (and in The Doctor's Diet).

Unsaturated fats fall into two categories: monounsaturated and polyunsaturated. They're each good for your health. Monounsaturated fats and polyunsaturated fats both help reduce heart disease risk by improving cholesterol levels. They also help stabilize blood sugar. Polyunsaturated fats go a step further and actually seem to reduce risk of type 2 diabetes.

Two main kinds of polyunsaturated fats are omega-3 and omega-6 fatty acids. It's easy to confuse these two omegas, but they have different qualities. Both are essential to good health and contribute to many body functions, including blood clotting, brain health, and heart health. They're referred to as "essential" fatty acids because, since our bodies can't manufacture them, it's essential that we get them from foods.

✚ Omega-3 fatty acids, which reduce systemic inflammation, may play a part in protecting against cancer, inflammatory diseases, autoimmune diseases, and arthritis.

✚ Omega-6 fatty acids are also healthful, but they work best when they're in good balance with omega-3 fatty acids. Most of us get plenty of (or too much) omega-6 fatty acids, since they're found in many vegetable oils, but not enough omega-3s. The Doctor's Diet helps get your omega fats in balance by focusing a bit more on foods with omega-3s, and a bit less on foods with omega-6s.

MORE ABOUT OMEGAS

There are three major omega-3 fatty acids: ALA (alpha-linolenic acid), EPA (eicosapentaenoic acid), and DHA (docosahexaenoic acid).

It's fairly easy to get ALA, which is found in walnuts, soybeans, spinach, and some other leafy greens, and vegetable oils such as canola, soybean, and olive. DHA and EPA are readily available in fish such as salmon, herring, sardines, and white tuna. DHA and EPA can also be found in some fortified foods such as milk, bread, juice, and yogurt. (Read labels to find out which brands are fortified.)

Omega-3s are so important to good health that I think everyone should eat omega-3-rich foods every day. Fish is such a good source of omega-3s that I advise people who don't eat fish to consider taking fish oil supplements. Talk with your doctor before you do, because they can affect other medications you take, such as medications for high blood pressure and blood clotting. There's still a lot of research that needs to be done.

SOURCES OF MONOUNSATURATED FAT

+ Nuts and nut oils
+ Peanuts and peanut oil
  (peanuts are technically
  not nuts, but legumes)
+ Seeds
+ Avocado
+ Olive oil
+ Safflower oil (high oleic)
+ Vegetable oils, such as
  canola and sunflower

SOURCES OF OMEGA-6 POLYUNSATURATED FAT

+ Soybean oil
+ Corn oil
+ Safflower oil
+ Grapeseed oil
+ Sesame oil

SOURCES OF OMEGA-3 POLYUNSATURATED FAT

- Salmon
- Tuna
- Sardines
- Mackerel
- Shellfish

- Walnuts
- Flaxseed
- Canola oil
- Soybean oil
- Olive oil

THE AMAZING AVOCADO

Once thought of as little more than the main ingredient in guacamole, the avocado is actually so full of nutrients that it's sometimes referred to as the world's healthiest food. Not many days go by where I don't include avocados in my diet. There's a lot to love about avocados, which are the fruit of an evergreen grown in California, Latin America, and other warm climates.

Avocados are a great source of monounsaturated fat, which is a truly "good" fat, especially if you eat it in place of less-healthy fats.

They also contain about 20 essential nutrients, including fiber, vitamin K, folate, potassium, vitamin E, magnesium, vitamin C, vitamin B6, and significant amounts of antioxidants such as lutein, which helps lower risk of macular degeneration, an eye disease that can cause blindness.

Not only do they bring their own nutritional advantages to your table, but they magnify the good stuff in other foods as well. Avocados work as "nutrient boosters" that actually increase your body's ability to absorb the health-building compounds in foods paired with them, such as the antioxidants in spinach, carrots, tomatoes, and other vegetables. That's why it makes so much sense to add them to salads, dips, and other veggie-dense foods. Plus they taste great.

I love smartly made guacamole—I use it as a dip for vegetables and a spread for burritos and sandwiches. It's easy to whip up your own: simply peel and mash two or three avocados into a bowl and mix in some chopped red onion, minced garlic, chopped tomato, some cilantro, and the juice of a lime. If you like a spicy kick, mix in some cumin, chili powder, diced jalapeño peppers, or a splash of hot sauce.

But don't stop at guacamole—there are countless other ways to include avocado in your diet. Blend it into smoothies, toss it into salads, add it to tuna instead of mayonnaise, serve it sliced alongside baked poultry, dice it up and mix it into omelets or vegetable dishes, combine it with berries in a salad, puree it with olive oil and garlic for a tasty spread to use in place of butter—the possibilities really are endless.

A CHANGE IN THINKING

Change can be hard, especially when you've bought into a certain belief for a long time. But change is also part of life, and the better we can be at adapting to new lessons in life, the better.

That's how it is with fat. For a long time, the idea that all fat is bad was hammered into our heads. And it's true: some kinds of fat still belong in the "eat only rarely" column. But now we know that some kinds of dietary fat are actually good for us, and we need to be incorporating them in our daily eating plans.

Here's one of the things I love most about healthy fats: you can use them to make other foods taste better. That really comes in handy with veggies, which are the focus of our next Food Prescription.

Vegetables play a major role in The Doctor's Diet. They're included at lunch, dinner, and in snacks. You can even eat them at breakfast, blending them into smoothies or tucking them into scrambled eggs. On the STAT Plan, we focus on lower-calorie vegetables—remember, when you first get started, we want to kick-start weight loss STAT. During the RESTORE Plan, you have even more vegetable choices.

The most important reason to include veggies in your diet is your health. Vegetables are full of all kinds of nutrients that do all kinds of wonderful things for your body, from protecting your eyes, blood vessels, and heart to boosting your immune system, keeping cells healthy, and even helping your body fight off cancer.

But there's more—and this is a major deal for us because we're focusing not just on good health but on losing weight: vegetables are turning out to play a crucial part in weight loss. Studies show that people who eat more vegetables are way more likely to lose weight and maintain a healthy weight than those who eat fewer vegetables.

One of the main reasons for the veggie–weight loss connection is that vegetables are filling because they're packed with fiber. When you eat high-fiber foods, they take up more room and spend more time in your digestive system than low-fiber foods. All that bulk in your intestines activates hormones that tell your brain to put down your fork and stop eating—or to wait longer before you pick it up.

What's more, there's a lot of water in vegetables—snap a piece of celery in half and you'll likely get sprayed in the face with more than a few drops. The water in vegetables also helps with weight loss because, like fiber, it contributes bulk to your digestive system, filling your belly and adding to that full feeling you get when you've had enough to eat.

A MATTER OF DENSITY

It all comes down to this: foods such as non-starchy vegetables and lower-calorie fruits (like the ones recommended during the STAT Plan) simply do a better job than most other foods at filling you up.

Here's what's going on. Vegetables are considered to have low energy density—that is, you can eat a lot of them for a small number of calories. (In comparison, high energy–density foods such as brownies or cheese have a large number of calories relative to their weight or volume.) With low energy–density foods, you can simply eat more food than you can when you eat high energy–density foods.

Here's an example. Say you're going to have a snack that weighs in at 200 calories. For that number of calories, you can have a couple one-ounce squares of cheddar cheese, which is a high energy–density food. As anyone who's ever been to a cocktail party knows, two pieces of cheese go down quick. But if you choose 200 calories worth of salad, you can eat way more food. For the same number of calories, you can pile a bowl full of all kinds of greens and veggies—and you can even drizzle it with a bit of dressing made of olive oil and balsamic vinegar *and* add some cheese crumbles as well.

A few chunks of cheese or a big salad with some cheese crumbles—which do you think will fill you up more? No question, the salad, which is packed with fiber and water and is laced with hunger-busting (and heart-healthy) monounsaturated fat as well.

When you look at all the evidence, it makes a huge amount of sense: including vegetables at most (or all) of your meals is one of the best ways we know of to satisfy your appetite and help you lose weight. And, as a bonus, you get giant servings of nutrients, too!

LEARNING TO LOVE VEGETABLES

Some people love sitting down to a giant bowl of raw broccoli or steamed cauliflower. They enjoy nothing more than plain-old raw veggies. Unfortunately, I'm not one of those people. When I was growing up, vegetables were an afterthought, they usually came from a can, and they were often swimming in butter or sauce. So it's been something of an adjustment for me to learn to love veggies.

Although it didn't come naturally, I made the commitment to learn to like vegetables because I know how nutritionally valuable they are. Yeah, I could probably go days without eating anything green. But if I do, I know I'm missing out on fantastic nutrients. I'd probably start putting on weight, too, because my hunger would send me off in search of higher energy–density foods instead.

The secret to learning to love vegetables is all in the preparation. Give me a stalk of raw broccoli and I'm likely to frown; sauté some broccoli in a little olive oil and garlic and sprinkle it with a little fresh Parmesan cheese and I'll probably be nibbling at it before you even get it out of the pan. Same goes for roasting: I don't care much for raw or steamed squash, asparagus, or eggplant, but if those vegetables are tossed on the grill or roasted in the oven, I love them.

If you're not a born vegetable lover, try experimenting with different ways of cooking, such as sautéing, stir-frying, roasting, steaming, broiling, and grilling. You may be surprised by what a difference a new preparation technique makes.

 EVERY TIME YOU DO YOUR WEEKLY GROCERY SHOPPING, BUY ONE NEW VEGETABLE. YOU NEVER KNOW WHEN YOU MIGHT FIND A NEW FAVORITE.

FRUIT OR VEGGIE?

Technically, an avocado is a fruit. So are corn, cucumbers, peppers, pumpkins, squash, and tomatoes. But their savory flavor makes most people think of them as vegetables, so that's what we call them in The Doctor's Diet.

THE COMPOUNDS THAT GIVE VEGETABLES THEIR VIVID COLORS ALSO DELIVER SOME PRETTY AMAZING NUTRIENTS. SO DON'T JUST STICK TO THE SAME OLD VEGGIES—EAT FROM THE RAINBOW.

WHAT'S IN YOUR VEGETABLES?

NUTRIENT	BENEFIT	BEST VEGGIE SOURCE
Vitamin A	Helps keep eyes and skin healthy; protects against infection	Sweet potato, spinach, carrots, pumpkin, peppers
Vitamin C	Helps cuts and wounds heal; keeps teeth and gums healthy	Red peppers, green peppers, broccoli, Brussels sprouts, tomatoes
Potassium	Contributes to healthy blood pressure	Spinach, Swiss chard, mushrooms, kale, Brussels sprouts, zucchini
Iron	Needed for healthy blood and cells	Spinach
Folate	Protects unborn babies from spinal cord defects; contributes to heart health	Spinach, asparagus, Brussels sprouts, avocado, broccoli
Magnesium	Helps with bone and blood health	Spinach, broccoli, okra, avocado
Fiber	Helps lower risk of heart disease, type 2 diabetes, and obesity	Cauliflower, cabbage, leafy greens, celery, squash
Calcium	Important for healthy teeth, bones, and muscles	Turnip greens, kale, bok choy, broccoli

FAMILIES OF VEGETABLES

Vegetables are divided into different nutritional families; some are members of more than one family.

+ **Cruciferous vegetables:** arugula, bok choy, broccoli, Brussels sprouts, cabbage, cauliflower, collard greens, horseradish, kale, radishes, rutabaga, turnips, wasabi, watercress

+ **Dark-green vegetables:** bok choy, broccoli, collard greens, dark green leafy lettuce, kale, mesclun, mustard greens, romaine lettuce, spinach, turnip greens, watercress

+ **Red and orange vegetables:** acorn squash, butternut squash, carrots, Hubbard squash, pumpkin, red and orange peppers, sweet potatoes, tomatoes

+ **Starchy vegetables:** black-eyed peas (not dry), corn, field peas, fresh cowpeas, green bananas, green lima beans, green peas, plantains, potatoes, taro, water chestnuts

+ **Other kinds of vegetables:** artichokes, asparagus, avocado, bean sprouts, beets, celery, cucumbers, eggplant, green beans, green peppers, iceberg lettuce, mushrooms, okra, onions, turnips, wax beans, zucchini

PHYTOCHEMICALS, CAROTENOIDS, ANTIOXIDANTS—OH MY!

If your eyes start to glaze over when you read about the nutrients in foods, especially vegetables and fruits, don't worry; it's a completely normal reaction. Unless you studied biochemistry or nutrition, it's likely that words like isoflavones and polyphenols will go in one ear and out the other. That's OK.

You don't have to know what all of these things are—you just have to eat them, and that's easy if you fill your plate with a variety of plant foods, especially vegetables, fruits, and legumes.

In a nutshell, "phytochemical" is the name for the approximately 4,000 different chemical compounds produced by plants and found in various plant foods. Some you may have heard of include antioxidants, carotenoids, flavonoids, catechins, and anthocyanidins.

Carotenoids are the pigments that give many vegetables and fruits their bright colors—the orange in carrots, for example. Some carotenoids you may have heard of include alpha-carotene, beta-carotene, lutein, zeaxanthin, and lycopene.

Although we don't know the full story of how these phytochemicals work in the body, we do have enough evidence to suggest that they are darn good for us. For example:

✚ People who eat generous amounts of carotenoid-rich fruits and vegetables have lower rates of heart disease and some kinds of cancer.

✚ The lutein in green vegetables contributes to eye health and may help prevent the onset of macular degeneration, a major cause of vision loss in older adults.

✚ The lycopene in tomatoes, pink grapefruit, and red peppers helps with healing and may protect men from prostate cancer.

Supplement makers have separated out some carotenoids and other chemicals in fruits and vegetables into vitamin pills in hopes of creating supplements that are as good for us as vegetables. But so far, none of the supplements seem to be anywhere near as good as whole foods at combating disease—in fact, in a few studies, phytochemical supplements have actually raised the risk of certain diseases. That's probably because compounds in vegetables and fruits work synergistically with each other in ways that we don't yet understand.

Might researchers someday come up with pills that replace vegetables? Maybe—although I don't think it's likely to happen anytime soon. In the meantime, you can get powerful packages of disease-fighting nutrients simply by eating a variety of veggies.

BROCCOLI TO THE RESCUE

Many studies have found evidence to suggest that eating broccoli and other cruciferous vegetables lowers the risk of several types of cancer, including cancer of the bladder, breast, colon, liver, lung, and stomach. Brightly colored red, orange, and yellow vegetables also contain compounds that are believed to fight cancer, heart disease, and some kinds of eye diseases.

VEGGIES, VEGGIES EVERYWHERE

Eating a plate of vegetables or a bowl of salad are just two ways to get the vegetables you need. But there are some other convenient ways to include veggies in your diet that may sound more appealing, if you're like me and don't love plain veggies:

Slurp up veggie soup. It's amazingly easy to make vegetable soup from "scratch." Follow my Anytime Vegetable Soup recipe (see page 257), or go free-form: sauté some minced onion and garlic in a little olive oil, pour in a can or carton of low-sodium chicken or vegetable broth, toss in whatever fresh or frozen chopped vegetables you have lying around (carrots, celery, broccoli, spinach, zucchini, green beans, cabbage—you name it), and simmer until the vegetables are cooked to your liking—anywhere from 20 to 30 minutes, depending on what kind of vegetables you're using. During the last couple of minutes, add whatever mix-ins you like, such as fresh herbs, spices, a small dollop of Dijon mustard, any kind of cooked legumes (black beans, chickpeas, lentils), or tomato sauce. Serve with a sprinkle of freshly grated Parmesan cheese.

Not only is soup a delicious way to add vegetables to your diet, but it can actually help with weight loss, according to researchers at Penn State University. Several studies from there found that when participants ate low-calorie soup *before* having a lunch entrée, they reduced their total calorie intake at lunch (soup + entrée) by 20 percent, compared to when they did not eat soup.

Veg out your smoothie. Add greens such as spinach or kale to your favorite smoothie recipe. Greens add a tangy taste that is surprisingly good, but it may take some getting used to, so start with a small amount and work up from there.

Vegi-fy your omelets. On mornings when you choose to have eggs for breakfast, vegetables can turn ordinary scrambled eggs into a delicious omelet. Sauté chopped tomatoes, spinach, onions, peppers, mushrooms, or other finely chopped vegetables in a squirt of cooking spray for about a minute before adding whisked egg or egg whites; then cook as usual. This is one of my favorite ways to load up on veggies.

Veg out with juice. Although I'm not a huge fan of fruit juice, because it raises blood sugar quickly and has little to no fiber, I'm fine with 100 percent vegetable juices such as tomato juice and veggie juices made at home with juicers. You should still eat whole vegetables, but it's OK to replace one or two servings a day with veggie juice. Choose low-sodium versions, because there's quite a bit of salt in the full-sodium kinds.

Make fresh veggie salsa your go-to sauce. Most grocery stores sell fresh salsa, which is a delicious mix of tomatoes, onions, garlic, lime juice, and cilantro. Spoon it right from the container onto baked or grilled poultry or fish, scoop it onto salads, stir it into soups, and use it as a dip for cut-up vegetables. If you want to make your own fresh salsa, check out my Anytime Salsa recipe on page 258.

Q: IS IT OK FOR ME TO PUT SALT ON MY VEGGIES?

A: There's been a lot of controversy lately about whether salt is safe for health. For a long time we thought high intakes of salt caused health problems, but recently opinions are starting to change, and the research is all over the place. I think this is a topic we're going to be hearing a lot about in the next few years.

Until the evidence is clearer, my suggestion is that unless your doctor has told you to avoid salt and sodium, it's probably OK to use small amounts of it. But in general, I recommend that you limit salt use. We tend to get so much of it anyway in our American diet, and my gut feeling is that going light on salt is a better idea than having a lot of it.

IN A 2013 STUDY OF 71,000 SWEDISH ADULTS, PEOPLE WHO ATE AT LEAST THREE SERVINGS OF VEGETABLES DAILY LIVED 32 MONTHS LONGER THAN THOSE WHO NEVER ATE VEGETABLES.

VEGGIES ON YOUR PLATE

I don't want to go overboard here, but the fact is that vegetables are just about the healthiest foods out there. They may not be your favorite food—I admit, they're not always my first choice—but when you think about how packed they are with all kinds of nutrients and disease-fighting compounds, you have to love them. And when you look at the studies that associate vegetable eating with long-term weight loss and longer life, you can't argue with the fact that they belong on your plate.

If, like me, you don't have a natural love for veggies, use the ideas in this Food Prescription to sneak them into your meals. As long as they're somewhere—blended into a smoothie, tucked into an omelet, chopped into a salsa—you'll get all of their amazing health benefits and weight-loss boost.

And now, in the next Food Prescription, get ready for some great news about another occupant of your grocery store's produce aisle.

As you know, I feel pretty strongly that we should be cutting added sugar—sweeteners added to processed foods, beverages, baked goods, breakfast cereals, and other everyday staples—out of our diets as much as possible. All that added sugar is a huge contributing factor to weight gain and disease risk. But when I suggest staying away from sugar, I'm talking about the sweeteners added to foods, not the natural sugars in whole, healthy foods such as fruits.

Yes, I'm telling you to eat fruit.

I know I'm going to get some flak for this. Most of the diets being promoted these days tell you to stay away from most fruit because of the sugar it contains. They say you can't lose weight or break your sugar addiction if you keep eating fruit.

I heartily disagree with this line of thinking. Unless you have poorly controlled diabetes and your doctor tells you not to, there's simply no reason to stop eating fruit.

Listen, I'm all about healthy weight loss and breaking sugar addictions. But I simply don't believe that cutting out an entire group of very healthful foods—fruit—is a good idea. In fact, I think it's a terrible idea.

As I've said before, the reason that two-thirds of Americans are overweight or obese is not that we are eating too much fruit. It's because we're eating too much of everything else.

Obesity researchers back this up. They have found no link between fruit consumption and health problems. In fact, long-term studies looking at the eating habits of large numbers of people find that eating fruit is associated with lower body weight and a decreased risk of heart disease and other weight-related health problems.

The nutritional benefits of fruit make it an excellent part of a healthy diet. That's why The Doctor's Diet includes fruit every day.

I'm not telling you to go out and gorge on fruit—absolutely not. You can't eat it in unlimited quantities, or you won't lose any weight at all. But by including it in your meals in an intelligent, balanced way, you can get a windfall of nutrients without any downside at all. And most fruit tastes great to boot.

So, come on, let's head out to the farmer's market or grocery store. It's time to start eating fruit again.

WHAT'S SO GREAT ABOUT FRUIT?

Fruit contains a cornucopia of nutritional benefits. Here are some of them:

FILL UP WITHOUT FILLING OUT

Fruits are high in dietary fiber (soluble and insoluble). Since I've already explained this and I don't want to get into too-much-information territory here, suffice it to say that processed foods are digested quickly, but fruit and other high-fiber food stays in the digestive tract long enough to allow satiety hormones time to send your brain plenty of "I'm full" signals.

The fiber in fruit doesn't just keep hunger pangs at bay: studies show it helps lower the risk of heart disease, diabetes, and obesity. And it helps keep your bowels functioning normally. Unfortunately, fruit juice has most of the fiber removed (more on this later), which is why I always suggest eating whole fruit or blending whole fruit into a smoothie.

SWEET WITHOUT ADDING SUGAR

Fruit contains a natural sugar known as fructose. Although it is a kind of sugar, the fructose in whole fruit does not raise your blood sugar the way added sugar in processed foods does.

The sugar in fruit is far different from processed cane sugar, corn syrup, and other sweeteners added to soda, cookies, cakes, and just about every other processed food out there.

When you eat candy, for example, you experience a rapid blood sugar response as glucose is dumped into your bloodstream right away. But when you eat a piece of fruit, the fructose within it takes a while to have an effect on blood sugar because it's hidden away within the fruit's dietary fiber—basically a fibrous net of cell walls.

Because your body has to work hard to break down the dietary fiber in fruit, eating it slows down digestion, giving you a feeling of fullness that you are less likely to get from low-fiber foods. It also allows blood sugar to rise gradually rather than rapidly, as it does when you eat candy or other food with lots of added sugar.

GOOD FOR THE GUT

You may think of bacteria and other microbes as being "bad." Some are—for example, E. coli can be toxic and can make you very sick. But our intestines are full of "good" bacteria and other microorganisms that assist in digestion, boost our immune systems, keep us regular, and do lots of other good things. Eating fruit helps keep your intestinal flora healthy.

A BITE OF GOOD HEALTH

The huge range of vitamins, minerals, and antioxidants in fruit helps lower the risk of a variety of diseases, including cancer and heart disease. The potassium in certain fruits (including cantaloupe, papaya, bananas, oranges, and berries) can help lower blood pressure and contribute to bone and kidney health. The vitamin C in many fruits helps the immune system fight disease and heal wounds. Other nutrients in fruit benefit your body pretty much from head to toe, contributing to everything from brain fitness to the healthy appearance of your skin, hair, and nails.

IN THE SAME 2013 STUDY OF 71,000 SWEDISH ADULTS CITED EARLIER, PEOPLE WHO ATE AT LEAST ONE SERVING OF FRUIT DAILY LIVED 19 MONTHS LONGER THAN THOSE WHO NEVER ATE FRUIT.

YOUR FRUIT-LICIOUS LIST

There's more to fruit than apples, oranges, and bananas. The best way to get a wide range of nutrients is to eat a wide range of fruits. When you're at the grocery store or farmer's market, consider popping lots of different fruits into your basket, including:

- apricots
- blackberries
- blueberries
- cantaloupe melon
- cherries
- gooseberries
- grapefruit
- grapes
- honeydew melon
- kiwi fruit
- mangoes

- nectarines
- papaya
- peaches
- pears
- persimmons
- plums
- pomegranates (seeds)
- raspberries
- strawberries
- tangerines
- watermelon

Q: I HAVE TYPE 2 DIABETES. CAN I EAT FRUIT?

A: You'll want to check with your own doctor on this, but in general, diabetes health experts say it's good to include fruit in a healthy diabetes diet as long as it fits in to your daily carbohydrate limits. For example, the American Diabetes Association (ADA) encourages fruit consumption as part of its carbohydrate-counting method for managing blood glucose. It can be eaten in exchange for such other sources of carbohydrates in your meal plan as starches, grains, or dairy. Because fruits vary in their carbohydrate content, the ADA program recommends limiting portion sizes to 15 grams of carbohydrates—the equivalent of about 1 small piece of fresh fruit (4 ounces), ½ cup of frozen or canned fruit (without syrup or juice), ¾ to 1 cup of fresh berries or melon, or 2 tablespoons of dried fruit.

Q: IS DRIED FRUIT INCLUDED IN THE DOCTOR'S DIET?

A: Raisins, dates, and other dried fruits are not recommended in the STAT and RESTORE Plans, but they are part of the MAINTAIN Plan. Dried fruits contain a fair amount of concentrated sugar. They're still fruit, so they're a better choice than cookies, donuts, and other processed foods with added sugar. Although they're small, they're high in calories, so it's easy to eat too many.

THE BERRY BEST FRUITS

Berries are an important part of The Doctor's Diet. Blueberries, blackberries, strawberries, and raspberries are fantastic sources of a variety of antioxidants, which protect cells from damage and help fight disease. In fact, they have higher antioxidant levels than any other fresh fruits. (Apples, cherries, and plums also rank high on lists of foods with antioxidants.)

Antioxidants in berries are believed to help prevent some kinds of cancers, as well as protect the health of the heart, brain, eyes, and immune system. Berries are a great source of other nutrients as well—including fiber and vitamin C.

Berries stand out for another reason: they have less impact on blood sugar than most other fruits. If you have diabetes or your doctor has told you to keep an eye on your blood sugar, berries are a great choice because they have a low carbohydrate count and are low on the glycemic index (again, meaning they are low in sugar).

Go ahead and mix berries into whole-grain cereal and stir them into yogurt, but think out of the box as well—add them to salads, combine them with whole grains such as quinoa for a tasty side dish, or mash them up with a splash of olive oil, vinegar, and black pepper as a sweet-savory sauce for meat and fish.

Fresh berries in season taste best, but it's also fine to use frozen or canned berries (as long as they have no added sugar). I always keep a few bags of berries on hand in my freezer to toss into smoothies. You can also enjoy munching on frozen raspberries right out of the bag—they taste like raspberry sorbet!

Q: SHOULD I AVOID FRUIT JUICE?

A: Generally it's better to consume whole fruit than fruit juice. Even if fruit juice is made from 100 percent fruit, with no added sugar, drinking it still dumps a lot of sugar into your system all at once. Take orange juice, for example. Having an 8-ounce glass of orange juice pours 22 grams of sugar into your body. Without fiber to slow down absorption, that sugar gets into your bloodstream pretty quickly. If you eat an orange, however, you get about half the amount of natural sugar—plus, an orange contains a few grams of fiber, which slow down absorption of the orange's sugar into your blood. So my advice is to go light on fruit juice and to choose whole fruit instead. And if you do drink fruit juice, choose 100 percent juice rather than those fruit punch-type drinks, many of which have as much sugar as soda.

GO FOR WHOLE

Whole fruit is more filling than processed food, according to a 2009 study published in the journal *Appetite*. In the study, subjects consumed an apple, applesauce, or apple juice 15 minutes before eating a buffet lunch. Those who munched on apples consumed fewer calories at lunch and reported feeling fuller and more satiated than those who ate applesauce or drank apple juice.

FIXED ON FRUIT

So there you go. Not only do you have permission to start eating apples and berries and cherries and melon and peaches and all kinds of other fruit again. You have something even better than that: a prescription to start including these delicious foods in your diet—not just because they taste great and add valuable nutrients, but because they help with weight loss and can slash your risk of disease. What's not to love about that?

Nuts are one of my favorite foods—not just because they taste so good, but because they're so amazingly fantastic for health and weight loss. Almonds, cashews, peanuts, walnuts, hazelnuts, pistachios, Brazil nuts, pine nuts—I love them all.

I never go anywhere without a couple servings of these super-portable "fast foods"—and by fast foods, I mean that I can eat them in a hurry when I'm hungry between meals and tempted to snack on chips or other junk food.

Nuts find their way into many of my meals as well. For breakfast I'll drop chopped walnuts and blueberries into my yogurt, mix slivered almonds into my oatmeal, or spread pure almond butter on whole-grain toast, an apple, or a banana. At lunch I'll sprinkle pecans or pine nuts on salads, and at dinner I enjoy peanuts mixed into stir-fries or blended with Thai spices into a sauce for poultry or fish.

I do keep an eye on my serving sizes, of course. Although nuts are terrifically healthy, they are also fairly high in calories. What's nice is that they are so satisfying that it really doesn't take many of them to take the edge off food cravings. In the afternoon, a handful goes a long way towards satisfying my hunger. And they fill me up for a while, so unlike other snacks, they leave me satiated enough that I can easily make it to dinner without thinking about food again.

THE PEANUT IS ACTUALLY A LEGUME RATHER THAN A TRUE NUT. BUT SINCE MOST OF US THINK OF PEANUTS AS BEING PART OF THE NUT FAMILY, THAT'S HOW WE'LL CATEGORIZE THEM IN THE DOCTOR'S DIET.

The doctor in me loves nuts even more than the hungry eater in me. Really big studies that look at people's food intake, disease risk, and death rates over long periods of time have found that people who eat nuts tend to live longer than those who don't. This doesn't surprise me because compounds in nuts help fight off several of the chronic diseases that land people in the hospital, including heart disease and diabetes.

There's also some evidence nuts—especially walnuts—may offer cancer protection as well, although there hasn't been a huge amount of research done into the effect on specific kinds of cancer.

Last but not least, nuts are an important weight-loss tool—which is really the number one reason that they're part of The Doctor's Diet. Nuts and nut butters are a very effective way to lose weight and keep it off permanently, so they're part of every phase of The Doctor's Diet.

I ask you: What's not to love about these portable little packets of nutrition and flavor? If you aren't eating nuts (and assuming you're not allergic to them), now's a really good time to start adding them to your diet.

WHY AM I NUTS ABOUT NUTS?

Some 20 years ago, researchers started to shine an intense light on nuts, looking to quantify their impact on our diets. Nuts are an integral part of the Mediterranean diet, which has been associated with some dramatic health benefits. (The Mediterranean diet is an eating pattern that focuses on fruits, vegetables, whole grains, nuts, legumes, seeds, herbs and spices, seafood, and olive oil, while incorporating some dairy foods and eggs and limiting sweets and red meat.)

Nuts have been the topic of many large studies in the United States, Europe, and elsewhere in the world. The results consistently point toward nuts being an important food for good health and weight loss.

For example, we recently heard about the results of PREDIMED, a Spanish study of 7,216 men and women ages 55 to 90 with elevated risk of heart disease. For about five years, the study compared the health of people who ate nuts with those who didn't eat nuts. The findings, published in 2013 in the journal *BMC Medicine*, showed that nut eaters were less likely to die during the study than non–nut eaters. Here are some specifics:

+ People who ate one to three servings of nuts (1 ounce, or 28 grams) each week were 29 percent less likely to die during the study period than those who ate no nuts.

+ People who ate three or more servings of nuts weekly were even less likely to die (39 percent) during the study than those who did not eat nuts.

+ The results are even better for heart disease and cancer: people in the study who ate three or more servings of nuts a week were 55 percent less likely to die from heart disease and 40 percent less likely to die from cancer.

+ Those who ate nuts had, on average, a smaller body mass index and waist size than those who didn't.

WHAT'S SO SPECIAL ABOUT NUTS?

Nuts have a lot of things going for them, health-wise, including the following:

Slimming power. Even though they're delicious and relatively high in fat, nuts actually help with weight loss. Take a look at the research on nuts and weight and you'll find that, to put it simply, people who eat nuts tend to weigh less than those who don't.

For example, a 2011 study of more than 120,000 men and women in the US published in the *New England Journal of Medicine* found that people who ate nuts gained noticeably less weight over the course of 20 years than those who didn't. Similarly, a 2007 study published in the journal *Obesity* showed that participants who ate nuts two or more times per week were 31 percent less likely to gain weight after 28 months than those who rarely ate nuts.

Other studies have shown that weight loss is more likely to succeed when people are following reduced-calorie diets. Subjects in these studies find they are better able to stick with their eating plans and lose weight if they include nuts in their diet. What it comes down to is this: a weight-loss diet is simply more filling, more palatable, and more enjoyable when it contains nuts.

Hunger zappers. Nuts are very filling—in fact, the combination of protein, fat, and fiber in nuts makes them one of the most filling foods out there. In nutrition studies, when researchers ask subjects to add nuts to their diet, the subjects tend to eat less of other foods even if the research-ers don't ask them to cut back. People who eat nuts feel full enough after eating them that they naturally skip eating other (often less-healthy) foods.

Nuts can be a real gift if you struggle with hunger pangs. The nutrition equation in nuts—protein + fiber + healthy fat—is a just-right hunger fighter that can satisfy your appetite for hours after you eat them.

How long do nuts stay with you? Longer than you might think, according to a 2013 study published in the *British Journal of Nutrition*. In this study, participants who had either 1.5 ounces of peanuts or 3 tablespoons of peanut butter (about a serving and a half) at breakfast reported that they had lower desire to eat for 8 to 12 hours after their morning meal compared with people who had no nuts at breakfast. (They had a high-carbohydrate breakfast instead.) Researchers looked at the study participants' blood and found that those who ate peanuts or peanut butter had higher levels of a hormone called peptide YY, which promotes fullness and satiety.

NUTS ARE VERY FILLING—IN FACT, THE COMBINATION OF PROTEIN, FAT, AND FIBER IN NUTS MAKES THEM ONE OF THE MOST FILLING FOODS OUT THERE.

Sugar balancers. One of the reasons nuts are such great hunger fighters is that their protein, fat, and fiber content all work together to keep blood sugar stable. Eat a sugary snack and your blood sugar will zoom up fast, spark a rush of insulin production, and then fall down rap-idly, triggering hunger, crankiness, and a craving for more sugary snacks. But eat a handful of nuts, which are very low on the glycemic index, and your blood sugar will rise slowly, eliciting a reasonable and stable insulin response, and then fall gradually, without all the cravings, hunger pangs, and nutritional drama of a sweet snack.

Over time, the blood sugar stability promoted by nuts seems like it may help lower the risk of developing type 2 diabetes. And in people with diabetes, replacing high-carbohydrate foods with nuts can help keep blood sugar in control. In fact, a 2011 study published in the journal *Diabetes Care* found that people with diabetes who replaced high-carb foods in their diet with two ounces a day of nuts saw significant decreases in tests of HbA1c, which are used to monitor long-term blood sugar control.

In the Nurses' Health Study, a large, long-term study of women's health, eating an ounce of nuts five or more times a week was associated with a 27 percent decrease in developing type 2 diabetes.

Fiber phenoms. Nuts contain anywhere from 2 to 3 grams of fiber per 1 ounce (28 gram) serving. Not only does fiber fill you up, but eating a high-fiber diet (21 to 25 grams daily for women, 30 to 38 grams daily for men) is associated with successful weight loss, heart health, lower diabetes rates, lower risk of some kinds of cancer, and an overall increase in digestive health.

Protein shell-out. Protein helps satiate your hunger and plays a role in successful weight loss. A serving of nuts contains about 8 grams of protein.

Just what the cardiologist ordered. Nuts improve your blood lipid profile—which means they help lower your total cholesterol, help bring down LDL ("bad") cholesterol, reduce triglycerides, and raise HDL ("good") cholesterol. Four large studies that followed the health of over 160,000 men and women showed that eating about 1 ounce of peanuts daily cut the risk of heart disease in half. That's a huge benefit!

Why do nuts help with heart health? We don't know all the reasons, but we do know a few. Some nuts, such as peanuts, are high in a compound called arginine, which can help open blood vessels and allow blood to flow more easily. Walnuts contain especially high levels of alpha-linolenic acid, which appears to help blood vessel walls increase their elasticity. (In people with heart disease, blood vessels can get stiff, hard, and inflexible.)

In the PREDIMED study I mentioned earlier, people who ate primarily walnuts had even lower rates of death from heart disease and cancer than people who ate other kinds of nuts.

Source of "good" fat. Nuts are a wonderful source of healthy fats. All nuts contain monounsaturated fats, and walnuts provide omega-3 fatty acids (which, as previously mentioned, are also found in salmon and other fatty fish). These fats contribute to heart health, help keep blood sugar stable, and may lower the risk of type 2 diabetes.

Nutty nutrients. Although different kinds of nuts have slightly different nutrient profiles, they generally are a good source of calcium, magnesium, potassium, vitamin E, and folate. Several of these nutrients, especially magnesium, potassium, and folate, are known to play a big role in heart health. They also provide a range of disease-fighting phytochemicals, such as phenolic acids, polyphenols, and phytosterols.

NUTS FOR KIDS

Nuts are great for children as well as adults. In a 2013 study of sixth-graders, those who ate peanuts at least once per week were less likely than non–nut eaters to be overweight or obese. They also had lower levels of total blood cholesterol and higher intakes of vitamin E, fiber, potassium, and magnesium.

SHOPPING FOR NUTS

When it comes to choosing nuts to include in The Doctor's Diet meal plans, here are some guidelines to keep in mind:

+ Choose raw nuts over roasted nuts. Scientists have found that the roasting process destroys some of the antioxidants and other nutrients in nuts.

+ Choose unsalted (or low-salt) nuts over salted nuts. You just don't need all the sodium in heavily salted nuts. At first you may balk at the salt-free taste, but before you know it your taste buds will adjust and you'll be perfectly happy enjoying the nutty taste without a heavy dose of salt. There are usually plenty of lower-sodium versions to choose from.

+ Choose unsweetened nuts. Americans find a way to put sugar on nearly everything, including nuts. Check the label for added sugar, and watch out for nuts coated with honey, brown sugar, or any other sweetener.

✚ Buy nuts in amounts that will be eaten fairly quickly, because they can oxidize and develop an off taste if you keep them too long. (Raw nuts are especially prone to this.) And store nuts in a cool, dark place. Some people keep them in the refrigerator or freezer.

✚ Experiment with different kinds of nuts. Most of us rely primarily on peanuts. But nuts vary in their nutritional content and since peanuts are considered a legume, it's definitely worth expanding your nut repertoire to open you up to a wider variety of flavors and nutrients.

✚ Try walnuts. Walnuts contain a few things that other nuts don't, such as certain kinds of phytochemicals. They also seem to come out ahead of other nuts in studies of cancer prevention, although researchers aren't exactly sure why.

✚ Explore the world of nut butters. Everybody's had peanut butter, but what about almond butter, cashew butter, and pecan butter?

✚ Check out the appropriate section of your local grocery store, natural foods store, or online retailers for different kinds of nut butters. Check the label to make sure there's no sugar, added fats, or other ingredients mixed in. (To keep the oil in nut butters from separating, stir them well and then store them in the refrigerator.)

NUT ALLERGIES ARE COMMON, AND IF YOU ARE ALLERGIC TO NUTS YOU SHOULD STAY AWAY FROM THEM. ALSO BE RESPECTFUL AND AVOID EATING NUTS AROUND ANYONE WHO MAY BE ALLERGIC TO THEM, BECAUSE EXPOSURE CAN TRULY BE LIFE THREATENING.

Q: I'VE HEARD THAT SOME KINDS OF PEANUT BUTTER CONTAIN SUGAR. IS THAT TRUE?

A: Unfortunately, it is true—most of the well-known brands of commercially made peanut butter contain sugar. It's not a huge amount of sugar—only about three grams in a two-tablespoon serving—but that's about three-quarters of a teaspoon, and if you're eating peanut butter on a regular basis, that adds up to a lot of sugar. Many kinds of peanut butter also contain small amounts of hydrogenated vegetable oils, which help prevent the peanut oil and solids in peanuts from separating.

Most grocery stores carry several brands of "natural" peanut butter that contain neither added sugar nor hydrogenated fats. These do taste a bit different than the sugar-sweetened peanut butter you are used to eating, but most people find that once they get accustomed to the difference, they actually like the natural peanut butter better because it has a purer peanut taste. If you can make the switch to unsweetened peanut butter you'll be better off, because you'll be eating that much less sugar and that much more healthy peanut butter. And if you can't stand the natural kind, experiment until you find a peanut butter or nut butter that pleases your palate. I've tried some brands of nut butters that I absolutely hate, but the ones I like always leave me saying, "I can't believe this is actually healthy for me!"

The main reason nuts are such an important part of The Doctor's Diet is what they bring to the table in terms of weight loss. When you munch on nuts as part of a balanced eating plan, they fill you up, keep you satisfied, and give you the energy you need to keep on going with your day while cutting back on calories. It's a simple equation: eat nuts, feel less hungry. Now *that's* something to go nuts about!

When was the last time you ate beans? If you're like many Americans, you haven't had them in a while—only about one in seven of us eat them on any given day. I think this is a huge mistake, because beans and other legumes are an incredible food. They have pretty much everything we need to lose weight and restore health; plus they're inexpensive and easy to prepare.

Nutritionally, beans are like the Swiss Army knives of food—they do just about everything. They even help with weight loss, which makes them such a useful tool in The Doctor's Diet.

But beans are more than just useful little packages of nutrients. In the kitchen, just about everything you couple them with gets better. Although they're tasty on their own, they really shine when they're matched with other foods. That's because they're able to take on the flavors of anything you pair with them, from spicy chili peppers to fresh aromatic herbs to fragrant dried spices.

Say you've got a can of white beans. Sure, you can heat them up and eat them as is, mix them into soups, or toss them onto salads. But if you join them with a few other ingredients—including tastes from around the globe—you can transform them into some amazing dishes. In less time than it takes to grill a lamb chop, you can make beans the centerpiece of a meal.

BEANS: YOUR SECRET CULINARY WEAPON

✚ Mash them up with garlic, a drizzle of olive oil, a splash of lemon juice, and a sprinkle of fresh oregano, and you have a delicious Mediterranean dip for fresh vegetables.

✚ Toss them with avocado chunks, fresh salsa from your grocery store, and a squirt of lime, and you have the perfect Southern California side dish for grilled fish.

✚ Combine kidney beans and black beans with diced red onions, chopped jalapeños, cilantro, olive oil, and balsamic vinegar for a zesty Tex-Mex three-bean salad.

✦ Lightly sauté them with garlic, fresh rosemary, and baby spinach for a flavorful Northern Italian sidekick to grilled chicken breasts.

✦ Stir them into tomato sauce flavored with mustard seed, cumin, coriander, chili powder, and turmeric for a distinctive Southeast Asian curry.

✦ Simmer lentils with canned or boxed vegetable broth, chopped vegetables (celery, carrots, onions), canned diced tomatoes, fresh ginger, paprika, saffron, and turmeric for a hearty Moroccan-inspired lentil stew.

✦ Turn everyday vegetable soup into a Tuscan specialty by mixing in kidney beans, garlic, chopped zucchini, and fresh basil.

I don't know about you, but my mouth is watering just thinking about all of those incredible meals. In fact, I think I'll make that curry for dinner tonight.

If you're still not convinced that legumes belong on your table pretty regularly, keep reading. I'm so blown away by their nutritional power that I'm going to wow you with seven really great reasons to include them in your diet at least a few times a week.

REASON 1: THEY PUT WEIGHT LOSS ON THE FAST TRACK.

Legumes are packed with fiber. More studies than I can count have drawn a connection between high-fiber foods and weight loss. It's pretty simple: foods that are high in fiber fill you up, staying in your digestive system longer than other, more quickly digested foods. People who eat legumes are less hungry compared with people who eat low-fiber foods with the same amount of calories. Legume eaters also tend to consume fewer calories later in the day.

All this fullness translates to weight loss, as confirmed in a number of studies. For example, in a 2009 study published in the *Journal of Medicinal Food*, obese men following low-calorie diets lost about 50 percent more weight when their meal plans included legumes. And a 2008 analysis of nearly 1,500 people published in the *Journal of the American College of Nutrition* found that bean eaters had lower body weights and waist sizes than non–bean eaters. In fact, bean eaters were 22 percent less likely to be obese than those who didn't eat beans.

Legumes are stuffed with both soluble and insoluble fiber. Soluble fiber generally helps the heart, and insoluble fiber keeps food moving smoothly through the gut.

THE AVERAGE AMERICAN GETS ONLY 15 GRAMS OF FIBER DAILY—FAR SHORT OF THE 21 TO 25 GRAMS RECOMMENDED EVERY DAY FOR WOMEN AND THE 30 TO 38 GRAMS FOR MEN.

Here's a look at the fiber content of various kinds of legumes:

TYPE OF LEGUME (½ cup, cooked)	GRAMS OF FIBER
Navy beans	9.5
Kidney beans	8.1
Lentils	7.8
Black beans	7.5
Lima beans	6.6
White beans	6.3
Chickpeas	6.2
Great northern beans	6.2
Cowpeas	5.6
Soybeans (edamame)	5.2

As we've discussed, eating higher-protein meals and snacks can speed up your metabolism, weight loss, and fat burn. Protein is an important part of The Doctor's Diet Meal Plan Equation for weight loss.

But eating plenty of protein doesn't mean eating loads and loads of meat. As we discussed under Food Prescription #2, eating a protein-rich diet doesn't mean piling burgers, bacon, and all kinds of processed meats onto your plate at every meal. Eating legumes allows you to get the protein you need without overdosing on meat or emptying your wallet.

You don't have to become a vegetarian or vegan to see an impact on your health. Evidence of this comes from several places, including a 2012 study of more than 120,000 adults, which was published in the *Journal of the American Medical Association*. Looking at people's dietary habits over the course of several decades, the study found that people who substituted legumes for just one serving per day of meat were 10 percent less likely to die during the study period than those who didn't.

On The Doctor's Diet, you can choose legumes instead of meat whenever you want. I can tell you personally that this is a substitution I make most days. That's one of the great things about The Doctor's Diet: you can make the choices that are best for you.

Take a look at the protein content of several kinds of legumes:

TYPE OF LEGUME (½ cup, cooked)	GRAMS OF PROTEIN
Beans (black, kidney, white, etc.)	7–8
Lentils	9
Chickpeas	6
Hummus (¼ cup)	4–5

REASON #3: AS THE SAYING GOES, THEY REALLY ARE GOOD FOR YOUR HEART.

Legumes lower levels of LDL ("bad") cholesterol when their soluble fiber binds with fatty acids in the body. They also bring down harmful triglycerides and seem to have a beneficial effect on blood pressure—all of which helps cut your risk of developing heart disease.

TYPES OF LEGUMES

Beans: adzuki, black, fava, garbanzo (chickpeas), great northern, kidney, lima, mung, navy, pinto

Peas: split, yellow, green, black-eyed

Lentils: brown, green, red, or black

 FOR OPTIMAL HEALTH BENEFITS, AIM FOR AT LEAST THREE CUPS OF COOKED LEGUMES PER WEEK. MOST AMERICANS GET LESS THAN ONE CUP A WEEK.

REASON #4: THEY SLOW THINGS DOWN—IN A GOOD WAY.

When you eat legumes, their rich fiber content slows down digestion of carbohydrates and the conversion of carbohydrates to blood sugar. That means blood sugar and insulin levels rise and fall gradually after consuming legumes rather than shooting up and plummeting down. That helps diminish cravings and overeating and is especially important for people with insulin resistance, prediabetes, and diabetes.

A 2012 study published in the *Archives of Internal Medicine* showed that participants who ate a cup of legumes daily for three months saw significant decreases in the results of their HbA1c blood tests, which measure average levels of blood sugar over extended periods of time. A diet rich in whole grains also lowered HbA1c levels, but not as much as the legumes.

In China, a 2008 study of more than 64,000 middle-aged women published in the *American Journal of Clinical Nutrition* found that eating legumes was associated with a 38 percent lower risk of developing type 2 diabetes.

REASON #5: THEY CUT YOUR RISK OF CANCER.

Studies show that people who eat a high-fiber diet that includes ample amounts of legumes have lower rates of colorectal cancer. The insoluble fiber in beans helps keep bowels healthy in several ways: it balances pH levels, helps remove toxins from the intestines, and prevents cancer-causing microbes from causing trouble.

Legumes contain a variety of cancer-fighting phytochemicals as well, and studies under way are looking at legumes' impact on other kinds of cancer, such as cancer of the lungs or blood.

A PORTION OF UNCOOKED (DRY) BEANS USUALLY DOUBLES OR TRIPLES DURING COOKING, SO HALF A CUP OF DRY BEANS IS EQUAL TO APPROXIMATELY 1 TO 1½ CUPS OF COOKED BEANS.

REASON #6: LEGUMES ARE PACKED WITH NUTRIENTS.

Legumes contain several important vitamins and minerals, including iron, magnesium, zinc, folate, and calcium. These help keep your heart, blood, and bones healthy.

I know, it sounds like a pretty big promise to say that eating legumes will help you live longer. But that's exactly what researchers found in a 2004 study of 785 elderly people across the globe. The seven-year study, published in the *Asia Pacific Journal of Clinical Nutrition*, found that for every 20 gram (about 2 tablespoons) increase in daily legume intake, study subjects were about 8 percent less likely to die during the study period. No other food group showed such dramatic results.

THE 411 ON LEGUMES

+ Legumes come from plants whose seedpods split on two sides when they're ripe.

+ Beans, lentils, soybeans, and peas are all part of the legume family.

+ Beans and peas in the legume family are referred to as "dry" to differentiate them from string beans and green peas, vegetables that contain a different set of nutrients.

+ Technically, peanuts are a type of legume rather than tree nut. But nutritionally they are more like nuts than legumes, so The Doctor's Diet considers them part of the nut family.

WILD ABOUT HUMMUS

If you haven't tried hummus yet, I strongly recommend that you run out to the grocery store and pick some up. Hummus is a snack food that I really love.

Hummus is a dip or spread made from cooked, mashed chickpeas, crushed sesame seeds (a paste known as tahini), olive oil, garlic, lemon juice, and spices. Optional ingredients include roasted red peppers, olives, spinach, artichokes, extra garlic, roasted eggplant, avocado, and other vegetables. It originated in the Middle East, but today you can find it in most supermarkets and convenience stores. It's also pretty easy to make at home.

The best thing about hummus (other than its taste) is its nutritional content: a two-tablespoon serving has two grams of protein, one gram of fiber, and no saturated fat, trans fat, or cholesterol. Most kinds are gluten-free. I love hummus as a dip for fresh vegetables or whole-grain crackers and as a spread on sandwiches.

COOKING WITH LEGUMES

It's up to you to decide what kind of legumes to use—canned or bagged. Buying dry beans in a bag and cooking them yourself saves money and allows you to flavor them as you like during the preparation process. But it also takes time, and easy-to-use canned legumes have the same health benefits as the ones that you cook yourself. (Some kinds of legumes, such as lima beans, black-eyed peas, and soybeans are also available frozen.)

If you use canned beans, check the label for sodium. If your beans are salted, a quick rinse under cold water will remove most of the salt.

Dry beans cook best when they're presoaked. Soak them overnight in cold water, or try this quick-soak method: Place beans in a large pot and add two cups of water for every one cup of beans. Bring to a boil and cook for two to three minutes. Remove from heat and let the beans sit for one to four hours. Drain the beans, rinse them, and then cook in fresh water until tender—typically about 60 to 90 minutes, depending on the type of bean. (For extra flavor, throw in a yellow onion and a couple of bay leaves.) Cooked beans can be kept in the refrigerator for several days or frozen for several months.

Q: I'M WILLING TO EAT LEGUMES, BUT I HAVE TO ADMIT, THEY GIVE ME GAS. IS THERE A WAY TO PREVENT THIS?

A: Suddenly adding a lot of fiber to your diet can cause bloating and gas. The key is to add it in gradually—don't go from eating zero legumes today to eating two cups a day tomorrow. Increase your intake slowly, over the course of a couple of weeks. Other ways to prevent gas and bloating include soaking dried beans overnight and rinsing them before cooking (it removes some of the compounds that contribute to flatulence), choosing less-gassy legumes (lentils, black-eyed peas, azuki beans) and avoiding major gas producers (lima beans, pinto beans, navy beans) until your system adjusts, and chewing beans thoroughly before swallowing. If you cook bagged beans from scratch, toss ⅛ teaspoon of baking soda into the presoaking water; it's believed to make beans less gassy.

Everyone makes jokes about beans. But when you include beans and other legumes as part of your diet, you get the last laugh. While other people are making fun of them, you are getting an amazing bundle of fat-burning nutrients every time you eat them. Yeah, they may be the "musical fruit," as we jokingly referred to them in grade school. But once you start eating them regularly, the music tends to subside, allowing their fantastic health benefits to shine through.

And speaking of foods that we joked about in grade school, maybe you're old enough to remember those 1970s TV commercials for a not-so-popular food that allegedly helped keep people alive well past their nineties. We laughed when we watched these really ancient Russian farmers eating a food that many of us had never tasted. But today we know that those crazy old commercials were actually right on target—in fact, the food they recommended is actually my next Food Prescription.

I've always been a fan of yogurt, but my esteem turned to admiration in 2011 when Harvard School of Public Health researchers named yogurt as one of the two foods that are most associated with healthy long-term weight maintenance. (The other food is nuts.) Now, yogurt is one of my top go-to foods, and it holds an important spot in The Doctor's Diet as well.

Here's the deal: Researchers have been following the health of about 120,000 doctors and nurses for a couple of decades as part of three big studies at the Harvard School of Public Health. Every few years, the participants are asked all about their health, their food choices, their exercise routines, their weight, and all kinds of other stuff. Then, the researchers sift through tons of data and look for associations between the choices the participants have made over the years and their health and weight.

In the 2011 study, which was published in the *New England Journal of Medicine*, the researchers compared weight change among study subjects with the kinds of foods they routinely chose to eat.

Just so you know, even though the people in the Harvard studies are doctors and nurses, they are just as prone to gain weight over time as everyone else. During the previous four years, the study participants had gained an average of about 3.35 pounds, which corresponds pretty closely to the average pound-a-year gain among American adults.

Once they crunched all their data, the researchers discovered that the food choices the participants made had a big impact on their weight.

People who routinely ate potato chips, French fries, potatoes, sweets, desserts, and sugar-sweetened beverages packed on the most weight

THE HARVARD FOOD AND WEIGHT STUDIES ALSO SHOWED THAT PHYSICAL ACTIVITY AND TV VIEWING INFLUENCED CHANGES IN WEIGHT. ALSO, THOSE WHO SLEPT SIX TO EIGHT HOURS A NIGHT GAINED LESS WEIGHT THAN THOSE WHO SLEPT LESS THAN SIX OR MORE THAN EIGHT HOURS.

every year—no surprise there. But what stood out was that people who ate vegetables, whole grains, fruits, nuts, and yogurt actually *lost* weight during the study period. The biggest surprise of all (to me and the Harvard researchers) was that yogurt had the biggest association of all with weight loss in the study participants—and the more yogurt they ate, the more weight they lost.

WHAT'S YOUR SECRET?

Why would yogurt play such an active part in weight loss? The researchers don't know for sure, but one of their theories is that the active cultures and good bacteria in yogurt, which reduce inflammation and contribute to the health of your digestive system, also speed up weight loss and fat burn.

What exactly do I mean by "active cultures" in yogurt? These are actual living organisms. They include *Lactobacillus bulgaricus* and *Streptococcus thermophilus*, which convert pasteurized milk to yogurt through fermentation, as well as strains of *Lactobacillus acidophilus* (usually on yogurt labels, the word "lactobacillus" is abbreviated with just a capital L) and *Bifidobacterium animalis*, which is marketed under the trade name Bifidus. These living organisms in yogurt do good things in your digestive system.

Don't let the word "bacteria" frighten you. Even though we think of it as being something that causes illness, there are both good and bad bacteria in the world (and in our digestive systems). You don't have to worry about getting any bad bugs in your yogurt as long as it's made from pasteurized milk, as all major brands are.

It's also possible that yogurt's weight-fighting power comes from its protein and calcium. Protein promotes feelings of fullness, decreasing hunger and boosting satiety. And some studies suggest that calcium in dairy foods may do this as well.

It's also possible that yogurt eating is associated with some other kind of food choice or behavior that the Harvard studies didn't ascertain—although these studies are pretty thorough.

Personally, I don't need to know exactly why yogurt helps with weight loss. What matters to me is that it works—so I feel really good about eating it myself and making it part of The Doctor's Diet.

Beyond being a great food for weight loss, yogurt brings lots of other nutritional plusses to the party:

✚ **It's good for your bones.** Yogurt is a rich source of bone-building calcium and vitamin D, which is especially important for women, who have a higher risk than men of developing bone-thinning osteoporosis. Depending on the brand and serving size, yogurt delivers up to a third of your daily calcium need and 20 percent of your vitamin D. Find out exactly how much calcium and vitamin D are in your yogurt by reading the label.

✚ **It's packed with protein.** A cup of plain, low-fat yogurt has 12 grams of protein.

✚ **It's heart-healthy.** Studies suggest that eating yogurt may be associated with lower blood pressure, and it's often recommended as an important part of medically supervised antihypertensive eating plans.

✚ **It may be OK if you're lactose-intolerant and may improve GI health.** The live, active cultures in yogurt break down most of its lactose, a dairy carbohydrate that can cause bloating, gas, and other gastrointestinal disturbances in certain people.

BETTER THAN MILK?

There's lots of disagreement about whether milk is an important—or even necessary—part of a healthy diet. I admit there's a decent amount of evidence out there that people can get all of the calcium they need without drinking milk. But there's also plenty of evidence in favor of milk for those who enjoy it. My take on the milk debate is that if you like milk, it's worth keeping in your diet.

I do think yogurt has more going for it than milk. They both have protein, calcium, and vitamin D, but with yogurt you get all those great live, active cultures. And if you eat Greek yogurt, you get a lot more protein.

LOW-FAT VS. FULL-FAT DAIRY

There has been some debate lately about whether it's better to eat non-fat vs. full-fat yogurt or drink skim milk vs. whole milk. Most nutrition experts recommend skim milk, which is whole milk with all its fat skimmed off. But there is a growing number of people who think we should give whole milk a second look.

Here's why. When you pour skim milk on your cereal, you're getting a lot of carbohydrates and some protein. When you choose whole milk, you're getting the same amount of protein, but you also consume fewer carbohydrates because whole milk has more fat. Plus, you get a dose of appetite-curbing fat. True, that fat contains calories—about 50 more per cup of milk. But it also may fill you up more, allowing you to feel less hungry through the rest of the morning.

Another common argument against full-fat dairy milk is that the fat it contains is saturated. For years, organizations such as the American Heart Association have been telling us that full-fat dairy products such as whole milk raise heart disease risk. But as with red meat, new research is suggesting that when cows are allowed to graze on grass rather than eating highly processed, nutritionally deficient feed, their milk is more nutritious even when the fat is left in.

For example, a 2010 study published in the *American Journal of Clinical Nutrition* found that consuming full-fat dairy products from grass-fed cows may actually *lower* heart attack risk by as much as 50 percent.

If all this leaves you scratching your head, don't feel bad—I'm scratching mine, too. I'm going to continue to keep a close eye on the research on dairy. In the meantime, I'm going to go ahead and put a teaspoon of half-and-half into my coffee (instead of sugar), pour low-fat milk on my cereal, and eat non-fat Greek yogurt because it's what I enjoy. My recommendation for you is to go with what you like once you've reached your goal weight, but be conscious of calories and serving sizes if you go full-fat. The STAT and RESTORE Plans recommend low-fat dairy to keep calories low. But stay tuned as we learn more about this debate.

Q: I'VE HEARD SO MUCH ABOUT GREEK YOGURT. IS IT BETTER THAN THE USUAL YOGURT I SEE IN MY GROCERY STORE?

A: They're both good, but Greek yogurt may be superior for a few reasons. It's made differently than ordinary yogurt, so it contains about half the sugar and double the protein. Because of this, Greek yogurt tends to be tangier, creamier, and less sweet than ordinary yogurt. Greek yogurt is my go-to choice, and I sweeten it by adding fruit or a touch of honey.

YOGURT BUYING GUIDE

The number of yogurt choices has exploded in the past few years—you can get dizzy looking at all the yogurt options in your local supermarket. Here are some tips on making the healthiest picks:

✚ Look for live, active cultures. The beneficial bacteria in yogurt enhance digestion, improve nutrient absorption, boost the immune system, and inhibit the growth of harmful bacteria in the digestive system. Check yogurt container labels for the presence of cultures such as *L. bulgaricus*, *S. thermophilus*, *L. acidophilus*, *Bifidus* (again, a trade name for *Bifidobacterium animalis*), *L. casei* and *L. reuteri*. Some yogurt products are heat-treated after fermentation, which kills most of the beneficial active cultures found in the yogurt. So be sure your yogurt label lists "live, active cultures."

✚ **Skip the jam-like fruits.** Many "fruit" yogurts contain a highly sweetened fruit mixture that is really more like jam than actual fruit. It is loaded with sugar, and it turns a healthy food into an over-sweetened disgrace. If you like fruit in your yogurt, stir in your own fresh strawberries, raspberries, or chopped, pitted stone fruit (i.e., plums, cherries, peaches, etc.).

✚ **Stay away from the mix-ins.** Pretty much anything that comes in those little mix-in capsules attached to yogurt containers is full of sugar. If you like a little crunch in your yogurt, stir in your own chopped nuts.

✚ **Watch out for sugar.** Even the fruit-free varieties can be loaded with sugar—a cup of vanilla yogurt, for example, can contain several teaspoons of added sugar.

✚ **Watch out for artificial sweeteners.** To trim calories, some yogurts rely on aspartame and other sugar substitutes.

✚ **Retrain your palate.** The healthiest choice is plain, low-fat yogurt. If you're accustomed to overly sweet yogurt with lots of junk added in, you may not love plain yogurt at first. But as you progress on The Doctor's Diet—as you cut out super-sweet processed foods and increase your focus on whole, natural foods—your palate will change and you'll most likely find a new appreciation for the flavor of plain yogurt. And remember—you can always stir in your own add-ins (fruit, nuts, a little honey) for extra flavor and texture.

✚ **Don't get your kids hooked on "kid-gurt."** Some are terribly high in sugar and calories, and with mix-ins ranging from sweetened cereal to ground-up cookies, they're really just desserts disguised as health foods.

✚ **Be wary of fro-yo.** Frozen yogurt sounds healthy, but it often is only marginally better than ice cream. Depending on the brand and variety, fro-yo can be packed with sugar and fat. And it may contain few or none of the live, active cultures that make yogurt so beneficial. Be sure to read fro-yo labels carefully before you buy.

OTHER WAYS TO EAT YOGURT

It's not just for breakfast. You can include yogurt in healthy meals throughout the day:

✚ **Make a smoothie.** Yogurt's creamy texture makes it a perfect base for all kinds of smoothies.

✚ **Whip up a dip.** Mix yogurt with chopped peeled cucumber, fresh dill, and minced garlic for a delicious vegetable dip.

✚ **Stir up a sauce.** Blend yogurt with olive oil, garlic, fresh lemon juice, and mint for an elegant sauce for fish or chicken.

✚ **Swirl it into soup.** A dollop of yogurt is a creamy change of pace in hearty vegetable- or bean-based soups such as black bean, lentil, and gazpacho.

✚ **Dress a salad.** Use yogurt in place of mayonnaise in your favorite salad dressings.

✚ **Serve it as a side.** Instead of the sour cream called for in many Tex-Mex foods, use Greek yogurt. It actually tastes better on many dishes than sour cream, and you get the added health benefit.

✚ **Build a parfait.** Create a luxe dessert by layering yogurt with fresh berries and chopped nuts in a fancy parfait glass.

There you have my 10 Food Prescriptions for optimal health. By following these recommendations, you'll put yourself on the path to a lower weight, a slimmer waist, a healthier body, and a longer life. I hope you'll take these prescriptions every bit as seriously as you would a prescription for a medicine or a medical treatment, because, as Hippocrates said, food really can be your medicine—provided you choose the healthiest foods.

Now that you understand how The Doctor's Diet is designed and you've had some time to follow the STAT Plan, I'll tell you about the next phase of my eating program: the RESTORE Plan.

PART THREE
THE DOCTOR'S DIET RESTORE PLAN

After kicking off your healthy new life with my 14-day STAT Plan, you're ready to move on to the next phase of The Doctor's Diet: the 14-day RESTORE Plan.

During your 14 days on the STAT Plan, you "stopped the bleeding" on your excess weight emergency. You began shedding pounds and burning fat.

By now you should be feeling some pleasant changes in both body and mind. Most people discover that being on the STAT Plan significantly lowers their cravings for sugar and high-fat junk foods. They also find their taste buds getting reset in such a way that they appreciate the natural taste of whole foods more than they have in years.

Now that you've completed the 14-day STAT Plan, overly sweet soft drinks and desserts that you recently enjoyed may taste way too sweet, and the salty, greasy snacks that you once craved may be far less appealing to you.

If you aren't seeing these changes, I'm guessing that your cravings and sugar addictions are so entrenched that you need a little more time to overcome them. Don't worry—if you follow the RESTORE Plan exactly as written, you should start noticing these changes very soon.

RESTORE ADDS EXCITING NEW ADDITIONS!

The RESTORE Plan is a natural outgrowth of the STAT Plan. RE-STORE builds on STAT by adding more flexibility and more choices.

Meal Plan Equations for breakfast, lunch, and dinner are the same for RESTORE as they are for STAT. However, you'll have a longer list of Fruits to choose from on the RESTORE Plan, in addition to STAT's apples, berries, and grapefruit.

To make things even more interesting, RESTORE expands the list of Whole Grains, allowing you to choose favorite foods such as whole-grain crackers, whole-grain pasta, and more.

Another big difference between STAT and RESTORE is in the daily Flex-Time Foods. With RESTORE, you get even more choices of foods to add into your daily menu plan. RESTORE gives you an additional Flex-Time Whole Grain choice (for a total of two per day), and an additional Healthy Fat (for a total of two per day).

Plus, RESTORE gives you one extra Snack Protein. That means instead of one daily snack, you can have two. I recommend that one of your snacks includes a Snack Protein and a RESTORE Fruit, and that one combines a Snack Protein and an Anytime Vegetable. This widens your snacking choices and gives you even more opportunities to eat healthy, life-supporting foods.

Finally, raise a glass to this part of the RESTORE Plan: each week, the plan makes room for two Alcohol-based Beverages, allowing you to enjoy an occasional cocktail or glass of wine or beer.

The goal of the RESTORE Plan is to continue allowing you to lose weight by eating reasonable amounts of tasty yet also the healthiest of foods. The emphasis will still be on weight loss, but with the RESTORE Plan, you'll add a wider variety of foods to your daily meal plans. Many of these come from the list of Food Prescriptions I recommended in the previous section.

The RESTORE Plan is designed to be followed for 14 days. After that, you'll either shift back to the STAT Plan for two weeks in order to continue losing weight, or if you've reached your goal, you'll move on to the lifelong MAINTAIN Plan.

Either way, you'll continue to restore optimal health, lower your risk of chronic diseases, and eat foods throughout the day that will help you live a longer, happier, healthier life.

THE RESTORE MEAL PLAN EQUATIONS

Use the following Meal Plan Equations to create your daily menus:

RESTORE BREAKFAST:
1 Breakfast Protein + 1 RESTORE Fruit

RESTORE LUNCH:
1 Main-Dish Protein + 2 or more Anytime Vegetables

RESTORE DINNER:
1 Main-Dish Protein + 2 or more Anytime Vegetables

RESTORE SNACK #1:
1 Snack Protein + 1 RESTORE Fruit

RESTORE SNACK #2:
1 Snack Protein + 1 or more Anytime Vegetables

DAILY FLEX-TIME FOODS:
Each day (at the meal or snack of your choice) enjoy these additional foods:

+ 2 Healthy Fats
+ 2 Whole Grains
+ 1 High-Density Vegetable

OPTIONAL:
+ 2 Alcohol-based Beverages (per week)

The basic guidelines for RESTORE are similar to those for STAT. Here's a quick review:

✚ **Stay on plan.** Follow the RESTORE Plan as closely as possible for best results. Use daily Meal Plan Equations to create your daily menus. Or follow my sample 14-day RESTORE menu.

✚ **Think ahead.** Save time tomorrow by planning your next day's meals today.

✚ **Size up your size.** When portions are given in a range—for example, Main Dish Proteins are three to four ounces—choose the low end of the range if you're smaller (under 5 feet 4 for women or under 5 feet 10 for men), older (over 50), or less active (under 30 minutes daily), and the high end of the range if you're tall, younger, or more active.

✚ **Get served.** Make sure you pay attention to serving sizes. Eating too much of even the healthiest foods slows weight loss.

✚ **Give protein a hand.** Use your palm as a measuring guide for a four-ounce serving of meat, fish, or poultry. Measure beans and lentils with a measuring cup.

✚ **Choose drinks that accelerate weight loss.** Avoid sweetened beverages and diet sodas. For now, enjoy plain water, coffee, green tea, black tea, sparkling water, or water flavored naturally with lemon juice or cucumber slices.

✚ **Keep it real.** Avoid artificial sweeteners of any kind. You may use small amounts of honey or light agave nectar syrup (up to a teaspoon a day) to sweeten certain foods.

✚ **Fill up with H_2O.** Continue to drink an eight-ounce glass of water before each meal and snack (and with your food, if you desire). Drink an additional two to four glasses of water throughout the day.

✚ **Scramble it up.** Continue to enjoy up to seven whole eggs per week (or three per week if you have heart disease or diabetes). Use olive oil cooking spray for scrambling or frying eggs.

✚ **Go low with dairy fat.** In the interest of keeping calories low, continue to stick with low-fat yogurt and milk.

✚ **Spice is nice.** Use healthy fresh or dried seasonings and herbs to liven up your foods.

✚ **Slip the skip.** It's best not to skip meals, especially breakfast.

✚ **Fill 'er up.** Continue to fill your plate, bowl, or mug with Anytime Vegetables, Anytime Vegetable Soup, and Anytime Garden Salad.

✚ **Make a date.** Stay on the RESTORE Plan for 14 days at a time. After that, you'll either go back to the STAT Plan or move on to the MAINTAIN Plan.

RESTORE FOOD LISTS

Food lists on RESTORE are the same as STAT, except that you'll have a wider selection of choices for Fruits and Whole Grains.

RESTORE FRUITS

✚ 1 medium apple *
✚ 1 medium grapefruit *
✚ 1 cup berries (raspberries, strawberries, blueberries, blackberries) *
✚ 1 small-medium (or ½ large) orange, pear, plum, or other fruit eaten out of hand
✚ 1 small (or ½ large) banana
✚ 1 cup chopped or sliced fresh fruit
✚ 1 cup grapes or melon balls
✚ 1 cup frozen fruit
✚ ½ cup canned fruit (packed in its own juice, but drain the juice before measuring)
✚ ¼ of a small melon

WHOLE GRAINS

✚ Whole-grain bread (1 slice) *
✚ Whole-grain English muffin (1 muffin) *
✚ Oatmeal—unsweetened (½ cup cooked or 1 ounce dry) *
✚ Whole-grain cold cereal—whole wheat, oats, or other whole grain listed as the first ingredient (1 cup) *
✚ Whole grains such as amaranth, barley, brown rice, buckwheat, bulgur, millet, quinoa (½ cup cooked)
✚ Whole-grain crackers (1 ounce)
✚ Whole-grain dinner roll (1 ounce)
✚ Popcorn (3 cups air-popped)
✚ Whole-grain pasta (½ cup cooked)
✚ Whole-grain tortillas (1 small)

ALCOHOL-BASED BEVERAGES

✚ 12 ounces beer
✚ 5 ounces wine
✚ 1½-ounce shot of hard liquor

* = STAT Plan food

 TO REVIEW FOOD LISTS FOR BREAKFAST PROTEINS, SNACK PROTEINS, MAIN-DISH PROTEINS, ANYTIME VEGETABLES, HIGH-DENSITY VEGETABLES, AND HEALTHY FATS, SEE PAGES 37–40.

With the RESTORE Plan, you can choose your own menu using my daily Meal Plan Equations. Or if you prefer, you can use the 14-day menu here. If you do, keep a few things in mind:

✚ Each day's menu includes daily Flex-Time Foods: 1 (additional) Snack Protein, 2 Whole Grains, 2 Healthy Fats, and 1 High-Density Vegetable.

✚ Plus, each weekly menu includes 2 Alcohol-based Beverages.

✚ Menu items in **bold** have recipes included at the end of this book.

✚ This menu is designed in a traditional breakfast-lunch-dinner style, with soups and salads at lunch and main-dish entrées at dinner. But if you'd like to switch it up, go right ahead—lunch and dinner on the RESTORE Plan use the same Meal Plan Equations.

G: Whole-Grain Flex-Time Food (2 daily)
F: Healthy Fat Flex-Time Food (2 daily)
V: High-Density Vegetable Flex-Time Food (1 daily)

	BREAKFAST	LUNCH	SNACK 1	SNACK 2	DINNER
DAY 1	**Nutty-Berry Smoothie (See page 239);** 1 whole-grain English muffin (G)	**Baby Spinach Salad (See page 244)** with **Versatile Vinaigrette (F) (See page 244);** 1 cup **Anytime Vegetable Soup (See page 257)**	1 cup yogurt; 1 cup blueberries	Handful of nuts; ½ small avocado, sliced (F); sliced red peppers	**Curried Tilapia (See page 260);** ½ cup cooked quinoa (G); ½ cup corn (V)
DAY 2	**Cheesy Broccoli Omelet (See page 241);** 1 cup sliced peaches; 1 slice of whole-grain toast (G)	**Lentil Soup (See page 253);** ½ small baked sweet potato (V)	Handful of almonds; 1 cup raspberries	1 ounce cheddar cheese; sliced carrots dipped in ¼ cup guacamole (F)	**Spaghetti Squash with Meat Sauce (See page 262);** whole-grain dinner roll (G); 1 tablespoon **Rosemary-Garlic Olive Oil Bread Dip (F) (See page 275)**
DAY 3	1 cup strawberries; 1 cup yogurt; ½ cup oatmeal (G)	**Minestrone Soup (See page 254); Anytime Garden Salad (See page 258)** with **Versatile Vinaigrette (F) (See page 244)**	½ cup cottage cheese; 1 cup sliced peaches; 3 cups air-popped popcorn (G)	Raw veggies dipped in 2 tablespoons hummus and ¼ cup guacamole (F)	**Baked Ginger-Marinated Pork (See page 265);** ½ cup baked sweet potato (V); **Garlic-Rosemary Mashed Cauliflower (See page 272)**

	BREAKFAST	LUNCH	SNACK 1	SNACK 2	DINNER
DAY 4	1 apple spread with 1 tablespoon nut butter; ½ cup oatmeal (G) made with water	**Tuna Romaine Salad (See page 245)** with ¼ cup guacamole (F) and **Versatile Vinaigrette (F) (See page 244)**	Handful of peanuts; 1 cup melon balls	Celery sticks spread with 1 tablespoon almond butter	**Garlic Shrimp (See page 261)**; ½ cup brown rice (G); ½ cup green lima beans (V); 5-ounce glass of red wine
DAY 5	**Banana-Egg Pancakes (See page 242)**	Hamburger patty with lettuce, sliced tomatoes, onions, pickles, and ½ avocado, sliced (F); whole-grain English muffin (G); 1 cup **Anytime Vegetable Soup (See page 257)**	**Nutty-Berry Smoothie (See page 239)**	Handful of walnuts; raw veggies dipped in ¼ cup guacamole (F)	**Baked Cod with Tomatoes (See page 260)**; ½ cup barley (G); **Mediterranean Lima Beans** (V) **(See page 274)**
DAY 6	1 fresh pear; 1 slice whole-grain toast (G) spread with 1 tablespoon nut butter	**Caesar Salad with Salmon (See page 249)** and **Garlic Croutons** (G) **(See page 250)** and **Versatile Vinaigrette** (F) **(See page 244)**	Handful of pumpkin seeds; 1 cup raspberries	1 cup milk; 1 cup **Anytime Vegetable Soup (See page 257)**	**Beef Stir-Fry (See page 268)**; **Anytime Garden Salad (See page 258)** with **Versatile Vinaigrette** (F) **(See page 244)**; ½ cup green peas (V)

	BREAKFAST	LUNCH	SNACK 1	SNACK 2	DINNER
DAY 7	1 cup berries; ½ cup oatmeal (G) made with water; 1 cup plain yogurt	**Tuna Bean Salad (See page 245)** with **Versatile Vinaigrette (F) (See page 244)**	1 ounce cheddar cheese; 1 apple; 1 ounce whole-grain crackers (G)	Sliced yellow peppers dipped in ¼ cup guacamole (F)	**Pork Kabobs (See page 264);** ½ cup mashed sweet potatoes (V); 5-ounce glass of white wine
DAY 8	**Berry Smoothie (See page 238);** ½ cup oatmeal made with water (G)	Sliced baked chicken breast; raw veggies with ½ cup fresh salsa and ¼ cup guacamole (F); ½ small baked sweet potato (V)	Handful of pistachios; 1 pear	Raw veggies dipped in 2 tablespoons hummus	**Beef Skillet Stew (see page 264);** ½ cup green peas (V); whole-grain dinner roll (G); **1 tablespoon Rosemary-Garlic Olive Oil Bread Dip** (F) **(see page 275)**
DAY 9	1 plum or orange; 1 cup whole-grain cold cereal (G) with 1 cup milk	**Greek Lentil Salad (See page 247)** with **Versatile Vinaigrette (F) (See page 244);** ½ small baked sweet potato (V)	1 cup yogurt; 1 plum	1 ounce cheddar cheese; sliced tomatoes	**Main-Dish Roast Beef Salad (See page 262);** ½ cup barley (G) sautéed in 1 tablespoon olive oil (F) with onions and garlic
DAY 10	1 small banana; **Spinach Omelet (See page 240);** ½ cup oatmeal made with water (G)	**Tex-Mex Salad** with **Versatile Vinaigrette (F) (See page 244)**	Hard-boiled egg sliced onto 1 ounce whole-grain crackers (G); 1 cup strawberries	Handful of almonds; sliced red peppers dipped in ¼ cup guacamole (F).	Baked salmon fillet; **Baked Sweet Potato Fries** (V) **(See page 275);** Roasted Eggplant (See page 272)

	BREAKFAST	LUNCH	SNACK 1	SNACK 2	DINNER
DAY 11	**Banana Smoothie (See page 238)**; ½ whole-grain English muffin (G)	**Turkey Black Bean Chili (See page 255)** topped with ½ small avocado, chopped (F)	1 cup yogurt; 1 cup raspberries	Handful of sunflower seeds; 1 cup **Anytime Vegetable Soup (See page 257)**	**Ratatouille (See page 270)**; ½ cup lima beans (V) ½ cup quinoa (G) drizzled with 1 tablespoon olive oil (F)
DAY 12	1 grapefruit; **Mushroom Omelet (See page 241)**; 1 slice whole-grain toast (G)	**Vegetable and Cheese Salad with Pecans (See page 248)** with **Versatile Vinaigrette (F) (See page 244)**	Sliced apple spread with 1 tablespoon nut butter	Raw veggies dipped in 2 tablespoons hummus and ¼ cup guacamole (F)	Grilled chicken breast; ½ cup mashed sweet potatoes (V); **Rosemary Spinach (See page 273)**; whole-grain dinner roll (G)
DAY 13	1 apple; ½ cup oatmeal (G) made with water, sprinkled with handful (½ ounce) of nuts	**Chef Salad (See page 250)** topped with ½ small avocado (F), sliced, with **Versatile Vinaigrette (F) (See page 244)**	**Banana Smoothie (See page 238)**	Celery spread with 1 tablespoon nut butter; 1 ounce whole-grain crackers (G)	1 cup **Anytime Vegetable Soup (See page 257)**; **Salsa Chicken (See page 266)** served over ½ cup baked mashed sweet potatoes (V); 12-ounce bottle of beer

	BREAKFAST	LUNCH	SNACK 1	SNACK 2	DINNER
DAY 14	1 grapefruit; **Mediterranean Skillet Scramble (See page 240);** ½ cup oatmeal (G) made with water	1 cup **Anytime Vegetable Soup (See page 257);** open-faced grilled chicken breast sandwich (on 1 slice whole-grain toast) (G) with lettuce and sliced tomatoes	**Berry Smoothie (See page 238)**	Raw veggies dipped in 2 tablespoons hummus and ¼ cup guacamole (F)	**Pork Stir-Fry (See page 268);** ½ cup water chestnuts (V); 1 cup broccoli slaw dressed with **Versatile Vinaigrette** (F) **(See page 244);** wine spritzer made with 5 ounces white wine and unsweetened seltzer

PART FOUR
SAVOR THE REWARDS: ENJOY EIGHT AMAZING WEIGHT-LOSS PAYOFFS

Weight loss is a major goal of The Doctor's Diet, because excess weight is a major health problem that can deal you a one-way ticket for a trip to the emergency room. But now that you've been following my eating plan for a few weeks, not only should you be losing weight, but you are likely to be experiencing some of the other great health benefits that can come your way when you eat right, exercise, and shed pounds.

That's right, everyone—it's payoff time!

You've been putting in the effort to follow my super-healthy eating plan. Now it's time for me to tell you about all of the many health payoffs that have already started in your body or that await you as you continue to follow The Doctor's Diet.

I want you to savor the payoffs of excellent health, because they really can change your life forever.

In this part of the book, I explain *how* all the smart choices you are making with The Doctor's Diet all work together to help you feel better, stronger, sexier, and healthier. I also give you a bunch of tips on ways to multiply the great benefits that your healthier diet is delivering.

I'm proud of you for getting this far. Even if you haven't started following The Doctor's Diet yet, I'm jazzed that you're reading about it—and maybe this section of the book will motivate you to get started! Either way, you've taken big steps toward lowering your weight and boosting your health.

Following The Doctor's Diet will deliver a bounty of health benefits to just about every part of your body. It really is amazing how your cells, tissues, and organs react to healthy living and weight loss—these are truly some of the best things you can do for yourself.

But there's more. Much more! Once the fantastic health benefits of following The Doctor's Diet begin to kick in, you're likely to start feeling younger, stronger, and sexier than you have in years. One of the best pay-offs of weight loss is that you feel just plain better in so many different ways.

When your body is weighed down by extra pounds, it suffers in so many ways. But when you shed that excess fat and weight, your body responds quickly and dramatically. Risk factors fall, health problems become less serious, stressed organs are revitalized, and your body starts functioning better and better.

When you start losing weight, you'll begin to feel better. You'll notice that your clothes fit better, you'll feel less flab around your middle, and you'll smile more when you catch a glance of yourself in the mirror. You'll have more energy to play with your kids or grandkids, and you'll feel less worn out and beat down at the end of the day.

And once people start noticing how much better you look? Well, I don't have to tell you how great that feels.

Just as weight loss makes you feel lighter and freer, your body without all that extra fat seems to relish its ability to perform in the ways in which it was designed to perform.

Let me give you an example. Your lungs' job is, very simply, to take in oxygen and release carbon dioxide. This happens automatically, and without fanfare, hundreds of times per hour and thousands of times per day. But if you have excess fat, especially around the rib cage, abdomen, neck, and chest, your airways and lungs have less room for air. Fat prevents the diaphragm from descending fully and the lungs from filling to capacity. This means your lungs and the pulmonary muscles around them have to work extra hard just to get you the oxygen you need.

Adding to this extra workload is the fact that every fat cell in your body uses oxygen—remember, fat cells are metabolically active, so part of the oxygen your lungs pull from every breath goes to your fat cells.

When you lose weight and fat, your lungs have less work to do—not only because there's more space for your chest to expand, but because you don't have as many fat cells making demands on your oxygen supplies. As weight goes down, so too do the risks and/or severity of lung conditions and diseases such as shortness of breath, asthma, chronic obstructive pulmonary disease (COPD), and obstructive sleep apnea. Without all that extra fat, your lungs have more freedom to do the work they were created to do.

Similar reactions occur throughout the body when weight goes down. Here are some other ways your body benefits from following The Doctor's Diet:

A BODY THAT WANTS TO GET UP AND DANCE

When you start shedding pounds, your joints will thank you because you'll be protecting yourself from arthritis.

Having excess fat not only raises your risk of developing arthritis, it can make it worse if you already have it. Among normal-weight people, 20 percent have arthritis, but that number shoots up to 33 percent for people who are obese.

People with osteoarthritis, which is the most common kind of arthritis, experience pain when cartilage in joints breaks down. Cartilage damage occurs for a few reasons, some of which (age and heredity) you can't control. But it's also caused by the amount of stress placed on joints. The more weight you're carrying around, the more strain on your joints, and the more likely it is for cartilage to wear down.

The knees and hips are most affected because they bear so much weight when you move around. The knees, for example, support four pounds of weight and pressure for every pound of body weight you carry. So if you're 50 pounds overweight, that's an extra 200 pounds of force your knees must support with every step you take.

But even joints that don't support large amounts of weight are affected by body fat. That's because it raises inflammation. As we discussed earlier, being overweight or obese can raise systemic inflammation, which can cause damage throughout the body. The joints are especially susceptible to inflammation, which contributes further to the risk of arthritis.

When you lose weight and cool down systemic inflammation, you protect yourself from arthritis in the hands, wrists, and other non-weight-bearing joints as well as the knees and hips. Having less fat not only takes physical pressure off your joints, but it lowers the joint-destroying inflammation going on within your entire body.

Rheumatoid arthritis, which is an autoimmune disease in which the body attacks its own joint tissue, may also be affected by weight. Fat cells produce chemicals called cytokines that inflame joints and may worsen rheumatoid arthritis; having less body fat and less inflammation means fewer joint-damaging cytokines and other troublesome chemicals floating around in the blood. Some studies have found that obesity raises the risk of developing rheumatoid arthritis by as much as 25 percent.

Finally, there's gout, which is a kind of painful inflammatory arthritis caused by a buildup of uric acid crystals in the joints—most often in the joint of the big toe. As the number of overweight people and obesity rates have gone up, so has the incidence of gout. People who are obese are 10 times more likely to get gout than those who are normal weight.

Uric acid forms when your body digests protein and some other kinds of food. It's your kidneys' job to dispose of uric acid in the urine, but kidneys don't always work as well as they should in people who are overweight or obese. If uric acid doesn't get dumped into urine by the kidneys, it can accumulate elsewhere in the body, causing gout.

As with other types of arthritis, gout responds well to weight loss. Losing even a small percentage of your body weight lowers uric acid levels and helps the kidneys function better.

DON'T LET ARTHRITIS STOP YOU

Having any kind of arthritis can make it harder for you to exercise. But don't let that get in your way: even with sore joints you can still find ways to be active. Swimming, water aerobics, stationary cycling, and walking are all good options for people with arthritis. Some community centers, hospitals, YMCAs, and health clubs offer fitness classes designed for people with arthritis. Even if it's hard to get moving at first, try to remember this: losing as little as 10 to 12 pounds can reduce pain and increase your ability to function. So hang in there, and before you know it you'll probably be feeling better!

THE CHANCES OF NEEDING KNEE-REPLACEMENT SURGERY ARE 8 TO 18 TIMES HIGHER FOR PEOPLE WHO ARE OBESE. LOSING WEIGHT DRAMATICALLY REDUCES THE STRAIN ON YOUR KNEES.

MORE FUN IN BED

Not surprisingly, people who lose weight report having better sex lives. There are a few reasons for this. For one thing, diabetes and uncontrolled blood sugar can reduce circulation to the genitals, leading to erectile dysfunction and problems with arousal and orgasm. Vaginal lubrication may be lower in women with excess weight. And for both men and women, weight can negatively impact self-image and feelings of sexiness. Weight loss helps address all of these issues.

Weight plays a part in fertility, too. Studies suggest that excess weight contributes to about one-quarter of all cases of female infertility. (The jury is still out on whether weight impacts a man's sperm count and sperm health, although if I had to bet on it, I'd say it does.) Researchers don't know exactly how weight lowers fertility, but when you consider the exquisite interplay of hormones required to produce a pregnancy, it seems likely that hormone imbalances triggered by excess fat cells could very well play a part. Extra weight can interfere with successful ovulation, and inflammation may add to the problem as well.

Once they're pregnant, obese women are also more likely to experience pregnancy complications such as miscarriage, gestational diabetes, preeclampsia, and problems with delivery.

Losing extra weight before you try to get pregnant not only boosts your chances of conceiving, but it raises the likelihood of having a problem-free pregnancy and a healthy, normal-weight baby.

Research is linking excess weight with memory loss, Alzheimer's disease, and other kinds of dementia. In fact, studies basically show that the more you weigh, the less-well your memory works. Being overweight raises the risk of Alzheimer's disease by 42 percent. Losing weight can help reduce that risk.

Scientists don't know for sure how weight and memory are connected, but here's what they do know. Having diabetes, high blood sugar, or high insulin can put the blood vessels in the brain at risk. Damaged blood vessels do a poor job of bringing oxygen to cells that need it. Healthy brain cells contribute to good memory, and without enough oxygen, brain cells suffer.

Like the rest of your body, your brain likes to have a steady supply of nicely oxygenated blood circulating through it at a healthy rate. You can help foster good circulation by—you guessed it—eating right, losing weight, and exercising.

Systemic inflammation also can harm the brain. As you know, inflammation levels can go up in overweight and obese people because fat cells produce pro-inflammatory chemicals.

LIGHTER WEIGHT, HEAVIER WALLET

Here's another great payoff people see when they lose weight: lower doctor bills. Medical costs for obese people are an average of $1,429 higher per year than they are for normal-weight people, according to the Centers for Disease Control and Prevention.

Once you start dropping pounds and boosting your health with The Doctor's Diet, you'll begin to discover a new you. An improved you. A stronger you. A sexier you. We only have one chance to ride the merry-go-round of life—why not make ourselves the best we can be so we can enjoy the ride?

Next on our list of amazing weight-loss payoffs is a change in blood sugar that could potentially save your life. You'll definitely want to read about that!

You're following The Doctor's Diet because you want results, right? And you probably love the idea of *fast* results. Hey, who wouldn't? Well, I can't promise you that you'll lose all your excess weight instantly with my eating plan and Food Prescriptions, but I can tell you that there's one measure of optimal health that you can literally change in minutes.

I'm not kidding. In just 15 to 30 minutes after starting The Doctor's Diet—the time it takes for your first meal to start digesting—your blood sugar can begin to improve. As you stick with my eating plan and start to lose excess weight, your blood sugar levels can get better and better. And as blood sugar levels come down on a regular, long-term basis, so too does the risk of developing type 2 diabetes, insulin resistance, and other blood sugar–related diseases.

When I talk about the amazing payoffs of following my eating plan, I talk about blood sugar control for two reasons. The first is that it's one of the most serious diet-related emergencies we face.

If you want to stay out of the emergency room—if you want to radically change your chances of dying of a diet-related chronic disease—getting blood sugar in control is one of the best places to begin.

But the second is way more exciting than the first one: the blood sugar emergency is one of the most potentially reversible problems out there. Yes, it literally is possible to start addressing your high blood sugar problems in as little as 15 minutes.

Blood sugar is one of our biggest weight-related health challenges. But, amazingly, it is also one of our most solvable. Controlling blood sugar is a health payoff that truly is within reach.

THE BENEFITS OF BALANCE

When I talk to people about diabetes, I'm amazed sometimes at how little they know about how amazingly destructive this disease can be. Maybe that's because it's so associated with the phrase "blood sugar," and we don't automatically comprehend that something as seemingly benign as sugar can have such deadly power. But if you were to spend a few hours in a hospital with some patients who have experienced the disastrous complications of diabetes, you would see how catastrophic a disease it can be.

I don't want to scare you, and I don't like the idea of using scare tactics to get you to pay attention to your blood sugar. But when blood sugar levels are too high for too long and diabetes progresses, the complications can be very debilitating.

One major complication is blindness. Uncontrolled blood sugar can be so damaging to the eyes that diabetes is the leading cause of blindness among adults in the United States.

Another complication is amputation of limbs. We think of limb amputation as being something that happens to soldiers on battlefields—but diabetes causes far more limb amputations than wars. I can't tell you how sad it is to see someone you love lose a limb because of a diabetes-related infection or complication.

And of course, there's kidney failure and heart disease. If you have diabetes, you're very likely to get some kind of heart disease—in fact, 65 percent of people with diabetes actually die from heart disease or stroke. Believe me, I see this in the emergency room—when a heart attack victim is wheeled into the ER, there's a pretty good chance that person has—or had, in the case of those who don't make it—diabetes.

Enough of the doom and gloom—I don't want to bum you out here. I want to celebrate the fact that by following The Doctor's Diet, you're taking steps away from the ER. Remember what I told you in the beginning of the chapter: within as little as 15 minutes of starting my eating plan, you're on your way to better blood sugar control. Nice!

LOWER WEIGHT, LOWER RISK

Excess weight is the single most significant risk factor for type 2 diabetes. If you're overweight, your chances of developing the disease are multiplied by seven. It's even worse if you're obese—then you're 20 to 40 times more likely to get diabetes. Those are very dangerous odds!

Listen, I know that blood sugar may not be high on your list of fa-vorite things to think about. But it really is important to understand how blood sugar works. Once you understand it, you can take steps to keep it under control, and that's important, because the number of people with out-of-control blood sugar in the United States is growing at a stagger-ing rate.

Stick with me for this quick explanation of blood sugar. Just as our cars need fuel to keep moving, so do our bodies. For us, food is fuel—it delivers the energy we need to stay alive, and it gives our cells, tissues, and organs the power they need to perform the jobs they're designed to do. Without the energy we get from food, our hearts can't beat, our kidneys can't filter impurities from our blood, our immune system can't protect us from disease—you get the idea.

Cells and organs can't use food in the form in which we eat it. Our bodies need to process our food into a type of fuel that can enter our cells and energize them. This fuel is called blood glucose, or blood sugar. When you eat food, your body immediately begins to digest it, or pull it apart into components that can be used by your body. Carbohydrates (sugars and starches) in food are broken down into glucose, which is a very simple kind of sugar that can enter your bloodstream and travel to where it is needed to provide energy.

Glucose needs help getting into your cells—it can't gain entry with-out the help of insulin, a hormone produced by your pancreas. Think of insulin as a bouncer at a hot nightclub: glucose can't get into cells unless insulin, the cellular bouncer, pulls back the cell's velvet rope and allows the glucose to join the party.

In healthy people, this entire process takes place without a hitch. You eat, your digestive enzymes break down carbs into glucose, your pancreas releases insulin into your blood, the insulin ushers glucose into your cells, and your cells have the energy they need to do everything they need to do. Case closed.

But this process can hit some major life-threatening road bumps.

Your body's goal is to keep everything in the food-fuel equation in balance. It does so by constantly monitoring blood sugar and fine-tuning insulin production in response. When blood sugar is high, a healthy body produces more insulin. When it's low, a healthy body shuts off insulin production. It's a complex back-and-forth that goes on constantly as your body seeks to keep blood glucose in perfect balance.

In certain people, though, insulin—the bouncer that determines whether glucose gains access to every cell in the body—loses its ability to do its job properly. Instead of perfectly orchestrating glucose's entry into cells, insulin allows glucose to build up in the blood. And having too much glucose in the blood leads to two problems.

First, when glucose can't get into the cells, they lose their fuel source and are starved of energy. Without the energy they need, cells struggle to function in a healthy way.

Second, when there's too much glucose in the blood—a situation referred to as high blood glucose or high blood sugar—all that extra glucose begins to cause damage throughout the body. The liver and muscles try to help out by taking some of the glucose from the blood and storing it away, but they can take only a limited amount. Despite their best effort, there's still too much glucose floating around in the blood.

Over time, all that extra glucose in the blood starts causing damage throughout the body. It harms blood vessels and nerves. It interferes with the ability of organs such as the kidneys and eyes to function well. It even causes problems in sexual organs.

All this blood sugar trouble results in a disease that I'm sure you're familiar with because so many Americans have it: diabetes.

WHY DOES INSULIN STOP WORKING?

So we know that blood sugar can get way too high because insulin starts failing at its job of ushering glucose from the blood to the cells, where it is needed for fuel. The question is: Why does insulin stop working? Why does the cellular bouncer start saying "no" to glucose?

One "big" answer is excess weight—especially excess belly fat around the waist. Being overweight or obese and having all that extra fat makes it harder for your cells to respond to insulin. Scientists believe the kind of fat that collects deep in the belly (called visceral fat) causes a pro-inflammatory response that makes insulin less effective. In a situation called insulin resistance, cells become increasingly resistant to the action of insulin.

In other words, insulin says, "Let the glucose in," and your cells say, "Huh?"

Your body responds to insulin resistance by producing even more insulin. Your pancreas, which is located just behind your stomach, starts churning out insulin at a higher and higher rate in an effort to get glucose out of your blood and into your cells. Remember, your body's goal is to keep blood glucose at an even level—not too much, not too little. Your pancreas starts working overtime to supply the insulin needed to get blood glucose in balance.

For a while, the pancreas can usually keep up with extra-high demand for insulin. But over time, as your body needs more and more insulin, the insulin factories in the pancreas fall behind. This is when type 2 diabetes develops. (Type 1 diabetes is a different kind of disease that is not associated with weight gain but instead occurs when the pancreas stops producing insulin altogether.)

OTHER CAUSES OF INSULIN RESISTANCE

In addition to excess weight, several other things can contribute to insulin resistance:

✚ Inactivity
✚ Cigarette smoking
✚ Sleep problems, such as sleep apnea (more on that in Payoff #5)
✚ Steroid use
✚ Stress
✚ Certain medications, such as diuretics for high blood pressure

Insulin resistance, high blood sugar, and type 2 diabetes don't develop overnight. Most people have insulin resistance and high blood sugar for many years before their doctors officially diagnose type 2 diabetes. That's not surprising, since these conditions usually have no noticeable symptoms.

High blood sugar and insulin resistance start slowly, build up gradually, and only become type 2 diabetes when they hit a certain tipping point and you actually develop diabetes.

That build-up time actually has a name—prediabetes. Makes sense, right?

Prediabetes is a condition in which blood glucose is higher than it should be, but not quite high enough to be labeled type 2 diabetes. People with prediabetes are definitely on the road to developing type 2 diabetes. In fact, if they don't make lifestyle changes like the ones you're making as part of The Doctor's Diet, most people with prediabetes eventually get full-blown type 2 diabetes.

Scary and depressing? Sure, especially if you are one of the 79 million American adults who have prediabetes. But hang on for some great news. Prediabetes isn't a disease; it's a warning sign—a giant orange warning sign. If you find out you have prediabetes, you still have more than a fighting chance, because prediabetes is amazingly reversible. Simply by losing weight and making some other very doable changes to your lifestyle, you can protect yourself from type 2 diabetes even if you're already close to developing it.

That's right: research has shown that by losing weight and increasing physical activity, people with prediabetes can actually prevent or delay the condition from progressing to diabetes.

RESEARCH THAT KNOCKED MY SOCKS OFF

Here's how we know the extent to which prediabetes is reversible. More than a decade ago, researchers set out to look for ways to head off type 2 diabetes in people who were on their way to developing it. They launched a major study called the Diabetes Prevention Program (DPP).

Researchers divided more than 3,000 participants in 27 locations around the US into three groups:

✚ Group 1 made changes in their diets and activity levels.

✚ Group 2 made no changes to their diets. Instead, they took twice-daily doses of metformin, a diabetes drug.

✚ Group 3, the control group, did neither.

This is what the researchers found: after one year, the people in the diet and activity group—Group 1—slashed their risk of developing diabetes by 58 percent. That's a *huge* reduction in risk. Believe me, if you're a medical researcher and you discover something that cuts disease risk by 58 percent, you pop open a bottle of champagne, because it's a career-maker.

What's even more interesting is that the medication group—the people who took a drug that has for years been considered the first-line drug of choice for diabetes treatment—shaved diabetes risk by only 31 percent.

That means diet and activity were nearly *twice as effective* at warding off diabetes as the top-of-the-line diabetes medication.

But there's more, believe it or not. To me, this is the most amazing news of all. Remember I said the people in the study who lowered their diabetes risk did so by losing weight and increasing activity? When I first heard this, I figured they must have had to lose lots and lots of weight to get such incredible results—25 pounds, maybe even 50 or 100 pounds. But when I read the study, I was astounded when I learned the details: the average weight loss in Group 1 was just 5 percent to 7 percent of total weight.

That's right—just 5 percent to 7 percent of their body weight.

That means people who weighed 200 pounds dramatically slashed their diabetes risk by losing just 10 to 14 pounds.

I'm not saying it's easy to lose 5 to 7 percent of your weight. But it sure beats having to lose a ton of weight before you can even start to make a difference.

As for activity, the folks in Group 1 didn't start running marathons or hitting the gym five times a week. They simply added more activity to their lives. They walked, gardened, danced, swam, and got up off their butts for about 30 minutes a day, five days a week.

I can't tell you how exciting this is. If you are overweight or obese and have prediabetes, you have the power to turn your health around. Not by losing an impossible amount of weight, becoming a star athlete, or popping pills for the rest of your life. You can do it by making some reasonable changes in your diet and adding more activity to your life.

You can do this. I know you can.

WALK AWAY FROM HIGH BLOOD SUGAR

Activity is a great way to get blood sugar in control. When you're active, your muscles use their stored glucose for fuel and replace what they've burned with glucose from your blood. And the cells in active muscles are more sensitive to insulin than those in sedentary muscles. Activity is especially helpful after meals, when blood sugar levels tend to soar. Going for a walk nearly every day can lower the risk of type 2 diabetes by as much as 58 percent.

Q: SHOULD I BE TESTED FOR DIABETES OR PREDIABETES?

A: My answer to this question is an unequivocal yes. If you haven't had your blood sugar tested within the past couple years, it's time to roll up your sleeve and ask your doctor for a blood test. Of the more than 25 million Americans who have diabetes, 7 million don't know they have it. And who knows how many people with prediabetes don't know they have it. If your blood sugar is high, you and your doctor should know about it.

It's especially important to have a blood sugar test if you are overweight, inactive, over age 45, or if you have any risk factors for diabetes, such as:

✚ You have a parent or sibling with diabetes

✚ Your ethnic background has an elevated diabetes risk, such as African American, Alaska Native, American Indian, Asian American, Hispanic/Latino, or Pacific Islander American

✚ You had gestational diabetes during pregnancy or gave birth to a baby weighing more than nine pounds

✚ You have high blood pressure, abnormal cholesterol levels, or other heart disease risks

✚ You have polycystic ovary syndrome

✚ Your waist measures more than 35 inches if you're female or 40 inches if you're male

✚ You've ever had an abnormal blood sugar test

✚ You have other health problems, including diseases of the kidney or liver

LET'S TURN THIS EPIDEMIC AROUND!

We throw around the word "epidemic" a lot these days. You may think an epidemic is a disease that spreads from person to person, like the flu. You can't catch diabetes—but it truly is an epidemic, meaning way too many people have it and other blood sugar conditions. When it comes to diabetes, we really are talking about an epidemic, as you can see:

✚ 25.6 million Americans have diabetes

✚ 79 million Americans have prediabetes

It's a little hard to wrap your head around how many people that is. What it comes down to is this: nearly half of all Americans have diabetes or prediabetes. Nearly half! That breaks my heart, not only because type 2 diabetes is such a terrible disease, but because it's so preventable.

It's even worse for certain ethnic groups. Because of biological, genetic, cultural, and economic factors—known and unknown—some ethnic groups have even higher rates of diabetes. For example, compared to non-Hispanic whites, the risk of diagnosed diabetes is:

✚ 18 percent higher among Asian Americans

✚ 66 percent higher among Hispanics/Latinos

✚ 77 percent higher among non-Hispanic blacks

If you're in one of those high-risk ethnic groups, changing your diet and losing weight are even more of an emergency. But don't worry—diabetes doesn't have to be your destiny, even if the odds are against you. No matter what your risk, you can start taking steps today that will help protect you.

The writing is on the wall: if you're overweight, if you have prediabetes, or if you have other risk factors for diabetes, you can start making changes immediately that will help get your blood sugar in balance and lower your risk of developing diabetes.

Even if you have type 2 diabetes already, the changes I'm suggesting in The Doctor's Diet make a difference and can help prevent diabetes-related complications. In some cases, it can lower the amount of medication needed to help keep diabetes in control—if not eliminate your need for medicine altogether.

What it all comes down to is this: you have the power to make life-saving choices that will improve your blood sugar and protect you from diabetes. Even small changes can make a big difference. Diabetes doesn't have to control your life and destiny.

Plus, there's more: lowering blood sugar and diabetes risk also helps lower heart disease risk. That's your next big weight-loss payoff.

If you're like most people, you don't appreciate the work your heart does for you. Your heart works constantly, never taking a break for a nap, or a day off, or a vacation in Cancun. Every day it pumps about 100,000 times. Try squeezing your hand 100,000 times (or even 100 times!) and you'll start to respect the amount of work your heart does every minute of every day.

It's amazing. Using about the amount of pressure it would take you to squeeze a tennis ball, the muscles in the heart push your entire blood volume—about six quarts total—throughout your body three times every minute. In the course of an average lifetime, the heart beats about 2.5 billion times. I get tired just thinking about that!

We talk about our hearts breaking when a romance falls apart, but the fact is, your heart is one tough cookie. It started pumping blood about three or four weeks after you were conceived, and it's kept on ticking without a break ever since.

Considering the heart's role in human life, you'd think we would love it like crazy. You'd think we would all be doing our very best to take care of it—eat foods that help it stay healthy, do activities that help it stay strong, avoid habits that can harm its muscles and blood vessels. But, amazingly, most of us take our hearts for granted, making a lifetime of choices that not only fail to nurture hearts, but actually harm them.

And that breaks my heart, because heart disease is more than a statistic in my world. It's the harsh reality of having to say good-bye way too early after the death of a loved one.

EACH YEAR, HEART DISEASE CAUSES ONE IN FOUR DEATHS IN AMERICA (600,000 PEOPLE). IT IS THE LEADING CAUSE OF DEATH FOR BOTH MEN AND WOMEN.

Many of us don't truly appreciate and value our heart health until it's gone. I've seen this happen countless times in the emergency room. Patients—very often people who are overweight or obese—are rushed in with heart attacks, heart failure, cardiac arrest, you name it. Gasping for breath, clutching at their chests, they regret not taking better care of themselves. As the ER team tries to save them, patients bargain with God, promising that if they pull through, they'll join a gym, lose 50 pounds, and never smoke another cigarette or eat another bacon cheeseburger.

The fortunate patients survive, and the smart ones among them keep the promises they made while they fought for their life in the ER. They make a commitment to do everything they can to love their hearts and make them as healthy as possible.

I want you to make that commitment now, when you're reading a book rather than lying on a gurney in the ER begging your Maker to give you another chance. If you're overweight or obese, the writing is on the wall: there's a decent chance you'll end up in the ER fighting for your life if you don't put a new lifestyle plan in place now. Believe me—it's a heck of a lot better to make this decision now than when you're in the ER having your heart shocked back to life (if you're lucky) with a defibrillator.

By jumping right on to The Doctor's Diet, you've done the right thing. As the pounds fall off, you'll be lowering your chances of ending up in the ER with a fatal heart attack.

YOUR RESILIENT HEART

Lucky for us, our hearts tend to be pretty responsive when we start to take better care of them. Not all heart disease is reversible, of course. But many kinds are. And many risk factors can be reduced.

In a lot of cases, making lifestyle changes like the ones in The Doctor's Diet—improving your diet, losing weight, being active, getting blood sugar under control—can boost heart health. Simple changes truly can slow down, stop, or even reverse the course of some types of heart disease. Often, smart lifestyle choices actually do more for our hearts than the powerful medicines prescribed by cardiologists.

Whether you've got a diagnosed heart condition, you have risk factors for heart disease, or you've got a perfectly healthy heart that you'd like to keep that way, the lifestyle choices in The Doctor's Diet are just what the cardiologist ordered. (Of course, always check with your own doctor before you make any drastic changes to your daily regimen.)

As soon as you start following my program, your heart will feel the love. Almost instantly, changes will begin to occur in your body that will cut your risk of developing heart disease. Even minor improvements in your health can have a major impact on your heart, starting with four big benefits I describe below.

When it comes to your heart, a little care goes a very long way. So get ready to start showing the love that amazing little muscle in your chest deserves.

HEART LOVE BENEFIT #1: LOWER BLOOD PRESSURE

You probably know that having high blood pressure isn't good for your heart and blood vessels. But you may not know why, so I'll walk you through it.

Let's start with a definition: Blood pressure is the force your blood exerts as it pushes against the walls of your blood vessels. When your heart beats, it creates pressure that's needed to push blood through the many blood vessels (arteries, veins, and capillaries) throughout your body. The pressure actually consists of two forces:

+ **The top number:** The first force happens when blood pumps out of the heart and into the arteries. This is called the systolic force, and it's measured with the top number in a blood pressure reading.

+ **The bottom number:** The second happens during the very brief rest between heartbeats. This is called the diastolic force, and it's measured as the bottom number in a blood pressure reading.

Healthy blood vessels can handle normal amounts of blood

pressure—that's what they're designed to do. The walls of healthy blood vessels are flexible and muscular. They stretch like elastic when blood pushes against them.

Problems start when arteries begin to harden and blood pressure goes up, as it does when you gain excess weight, eat a poor diet, don't exercise, smoke, drink too much alcohol, or experience high levels of chronic stress. Genetics also play a part in whether you develop high blood pressure, which is also called hypertension.

One thing high pressure can do is cause microscopic tears in blood vessel walls. As these tears heal, thick scar tissue appears. This is called vascular scarring. Areas with vascular scarring attract plaque and other blood by-products, just as a branch that drops into a stream can collect leaves and other debris. When plaque gloms onto blood vessel walls, blood has less space to flow through.

Vascular scarring also raises the chances of blood clots forming in places where they shouldn't. These clots can cause strokes or heart attacks.

As plaque builds up and arteries get blocked, the heart has to work harder to push blood through narrow blood vessels. This can tax the heart because it's being asked to work harder than it is supposed to work. When vessels are blocked, the heart must exert more and more pressure to get blood where it needs to go, which raises blood pressure even more, not to mention the incredible strain it places on your heart.

Also when blood pressure is too high, weaker blood vessels can be stretched too far. This can create weak patches that are susceptible to rupturing, or breaking open. Ruptured blood vessels can cause hemorrhagic strokes and other catastrophes.

Once you start losing weight, there's a good chance you'll start to see your blood pressure go down. Even a small amount of weight loss can lower blood pressure. In fact, studies of overweight and obese middle-aged men and women with prehypertension (their blood pressure was elevated, but not high enough to be diagnosed as "high") have found that losing as little as 10 pounds lowered the participants' risk of developing high blood pressure by as much as 42 percent.

Exercise makes a big difference, too—I've seen patients start to whittle down their blood pressure simply by adding an enjoyable half hour a day of walking to their daily routines.

As with so many other weight-related health emergencies, some very small changes can make a big difference.

BLOOD PRESSURE: KNOW YOUR NUMBERS

BLOOD PRESSURE	SYSTOLIC (upper number) mm Hg		DIASTOLIC (lower number) mm Hg
Normal	Less than 120	*and*	Less than 80
Prehypertension	120–139	*or*	80–89
High blood pressure stage 1	140–159	*or*	90–99
High blood pressure stage 2	160 or higher	*or*	100 or higher
High blood pressure emergency stage	Higher than 180	*or*	Higher than 110

Source: American Heart Association

HEART LOVE BENEFIT #2: CLEANER BLOOD VESSELS

Heart disease can occur when blood vessels get clogged with cholesterol, which prevents oxygen-rich blood from getting to the heart. By following The Doctor's Diet, you're taking steps toward getting your cholesterol levels in order and unclogging blood vessels.

Cholesterol is a soft, waxy, fatty substance found in your blood and in all of your body's cells. Your body uses cholesterol to do some really important jobs, such as building cell walls, manufacturing certain hormones, and synthesizing vitamin D.

There are actually two classes of cholesterol: the good and the bad.

The "bad" cholesterol is low-density lipoprotein (LDL). LDL is the kind of cholesterol that gets lodged in blood vessels.

The "good" cholesterol is high-density lipoprotein (HDL). HDL actually helps clear cholesterol from the blood. Think of HDL as the sponge that runs through your blood sopping up "bad" cholesterol and carrying it to the liver for disposal.

Triglycerides are another kind of fat in the blood—they're not cholesterol, but they cause a similar kind of trouble as LDL, so they're usually thought of as being members of the cholesterol family. Together, cholesterol and triglycerides are referred to as blood lipids.

When it comes to cholesterol, your goal is to have less of the bad stuff (LDL and triglycerides) and more of the good stuff (HDL). The Doctor's Diet can help you meet that goal. The combination of weight loss, improved diet, and exercise can have a very positive impact on cholesterol levels. Many people who follow diets like mine see their cholesterol numbers improve dramatically.

BLOOD LIPIDS: KNOW YOUR NUMBERS

	IDEAL CHOLESTEROL LEVELS
Total cholesterol	Less than 200 mg/dL
LDL ("bad" cholesterol)	Less than 160 mg/dL for people who are at low risk for heart disease Less than 130 mg/dL for people at intermediate risk for heart disease
HDL ("good" cholesterol)	Women: 50 mg/dL or higher Men: 40 mg/dL or higher
Triglycerides	Less than 150 mg/dL

Source: American Heart Association

HEART LOVE BENEFIT #3: BETTER BLOOD SUGAR

We talked a lot about blood sugar earlier, so we don't have to go over it all again. But what does bear repeating is the fact that when blood sugar is high for long periods of time, blood vessels suffer. High blood sugar can cause your blood to get kind of sticky, which means you're more likely to form dangerous blockages and clots in your blood vessels.

When you follow The Doctor's Diet, you are taking giant steps to get blood sugar in control and lower your heart disease risk.

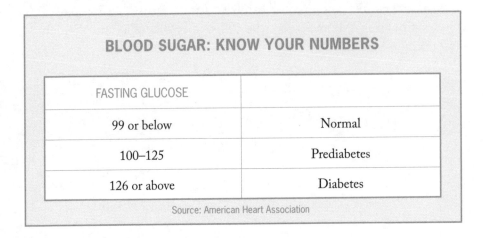

BLOOD SUGAR: KNOW YOUR NUMBERS

FASTING GLUCOSE	
99 or below	Normal
100–125	Prediabetes
126 or above	Diabetes

Source: American Heart Association

HEART LOVE BENEFIT #4: A SLIMMER BELLY

Let's face it: a slim belly is a sexy belly. But a slim belly is also a healthy belly—and that has nothing at all to do with how you look in a swimsuit.

I've already mentioned that deep belly fat (the kind you can't pinch), which is also called visceral fat, isn't just an unattractive spare tire sitting around your waist making your pants too tight. It's actually very metabolically active—which means it plays a part in the everyday business of running your body. Belly fat releases fatty acids into your blood, pumps out inflammatory agents, and produces hormones. Too much belly fat wreaks havoc on your heart.

The other reality about excess fat I've described is that it also requires a tremendous amount of oxygenated blood that must be pumped to it every minute of every day by your heart.

The more fat you have stored (in your belly and throughout your body), the harder your heart has to pump. All that extra pumping can actually cause your heart to enlarge in an unhealthy way—which is why obese people are likely to have larger-than-normal hearts.

Despite all this activity, belly fat contributes virtually nothing positive to your body (unless you're stranded on a desert island without food for a few months and need to live on the energy stored around your waist). Instead of being a helpful player in your body's physiological community, your visceral belly fat makes trouble for you and your heart by raising LDL cholesterol, triglycerides, blood sugar, and blood pressure.

As with most heart disease risk factors, you have tremendous power over your belly fat. The tools are at your disposal in this book because eating right, losing weight, and being active all help trim your waist. Cutting back on pro-inflammatory foods helps, too—we'll talk more about that later in the book. Luckily, a lot of overweight and obese people find that the fat around their belly is the first to go when they start to shed pounds.

Even if overall you're not carrying around much extra weight, having extra visceral belly fat greatly raises heart disease risk. I'm sure you've noticed relatively thin people with thick bellies—even they can benefit from trimming down at the waist.

BELLY FAT: KNOW YOUR NUMBERS

Having a large waist means you've probably got too much belly fat. Use the following measurements as your absolute maximum waistline:

+ Women: 35 inches or less
+ Men: 40 inches or less

To measure your waist, pull clothing away from your waist and use a flexible cloth tape measure. Starting at the top of your hip bone, wrap the tape measure around your body, level with your navel, keeping it parallel to the floor. Relax your breath and measure.

IF YOU NEED HELP QUITTING

If you smoke, there's no two ways about it: you've got to quit. I could fill the rest of this book and about 10 more books with the ways in which smoking damages your heart, lungs, brain, and every other part of your body. There is a lot of help available for people who want to quit. Start by talking with your primary care doctor, who should be able to refer you to smoking cessation resources in your area. You can also get help from these organizations:

✚ The American Lung Association:
www.lungusa.org/stop-smoking/
or (800) LUNG-USA (586-4872)

✚ The American Cancer Society:
www.cancer.org/healthy/
or (800) 227-2345

✚ Smokefree.gov:
www.smokefree.gov
or (877) 44U-QUIT (448-7848)

Q: I'M OBESE, BUT MY BLOOD PRESSURE, CHOLESTEROL, AND BLOOD SUGAR ARE FINE. SHOULD I STILL BE CONCERNED ABOUT HEART HEALTH?

A: Yes. Even otherwise healthy people who are obese have a higher risk of heart disease. A number of studies bear this out. A 2011 study published in the journal *Heart* found that obese men were significantly more likely to die from a heart attack even if they didn't have high blood pressure, high cholesterol, artery disease, or diabetes. The men actually had a 60 percent higher risk of dying from a heart attack than non-obese middle-aged men. It's not just men that are at risk: another study, published in

2002 in the *New England Journal of Medicine*, found that compared with normal-weight women, heart failure risk went up 34 percent in overweight women and 104 percent in obese women. So if you're overweight or obese and your heart health is good so far, that's great—but even so, excess weight does put you at risk.

CHANGE OF HEART

I love it that the human heart is so responsive to weight loss. Not all heart diseases are reversible, but many are, and when you start losing weight, your heart really can benefit!

But wait, there's more to this story. One of the reasons heart disease risk goes down with weight loss is that shedding fat lowers inflammation. Next, I'll tell you more about this exciting weight loss payoff.

WEIGHT-LOSS PAYOFF #4
A MAJOR COOL-DOWN OF
CHRONIC INFLAMMATION

Whenever I see video on television or the Internet of wildfires raging in states like California, Idaho, and Arizona, it reminds me of inflammation in the human body. When we are in control of it, fire is a huge gift to humans. Like fire, inflammation helps us in so many ways. But when it's out of control—when it burns for long periods of time—it can be a killer.

Inflammation goes up when we gain weight, eat certain foods, and live a sedentary lifestyle. But the good news is that we can bring it down. As soon as you started The Doctor's Diet, you began making changes that can cool down chronic inflammation. And as you lose weight, you'll spray even more cold water on chronic inflammation that's spreading like wildfire throughout your body.

FEEL THE HEAT

On the one hand, inflammation is an amazing biological response that we couldn't survive without. It's your immune system's response to danger. When something harmful invades your body and threatens it—for example, a virus or bacteria—your body's inflammation response turns up the heat in an effort to protect you from it.

Just as a police dispatcher sends officers to the scene of a crime, the immune system sends white blood cells to the area, along with several other kinds of inflammatory chemicals, including certain hormones and a kind of molecule called cytokines. Together they pummel the invader, fighting infection and helping your body to heal.

Think of this kind of inflammation—doctors refer to it as acute inflammation—as a controlled burn: things heat up for a while, but then they cool down again after everything is back on track.

On the other hand, when there's too much inflammation, it's not just the enemy that gets burned. Out-of-control, nonstop inflammation is like a wildfire, damaging healthy cells as well as invaders. Instead of bringing about healing, excess inflammation goes too far, harming the cells and tissues it's supposed to be helping. Rather than promoting health, your white blood cells, cytokines, and other inflammatory substances take on healthy cells and interfere with your body's ability to heal.

Having an inflammatory response that continues to simmer for a long time is called chronic inflammation. Eventually, long-term chronic inflammation can cause lots of harm to your body. It can damage organs such as the heart and the brain. It can interfere with cell division and contribute to the growth of tumor cells. It also messes with blood sugar levels and makes your cells less responsive to insulin.

Chronic inflammation has been linked to a wide range of diseases, including heart disease, stroke, cancer, diabetes, arthritis, and Alzheimer's. Pretty much all of the major killers in our society. Genetic factors also seem to play a part in inflammation.

In the case of heart disease, when the body perceives injuries to the heart's blood vessels caused in the way of high blood pressure, excess LDL cholesterol, and the buildup of plaque in blood vessels, it tries to heal itself by mounting an inflammatory response. Sadly, that response does more harm than good.

SOUND THE ALARM

There are lots of reasons why inflammation makes the jump from healing to hurting. The ones we're most concerned with in this book are the ones related to weight and food.

Eating a pro-inflammatory diet and having excess body weight and body fat are some of the major causes of chronic inflammation. That's because your body thinks of excess fat and unhealthy food as threats to your health.

Yes, you read that right: your body considers body fat and certain foods to be as dangerous as viruses, bacteria, and injuries, so it turns up its inflammatory response to a nonstop simmer in an effort to protect you from your own choices.

Fortunately, by improving your diet and losing excess fat, you can turn the heat down on inflammation. In doing so, you lower your risk of developing the many diseases associated with chronic inflammation—the very diseases that so often cause premature death and disability.

The Doctor's Diet is, at its core, an anti-inflammatory eating plan because it steers you away from pro-inflammatory foods and includes so many fantastic anti-inflammatory choices. Follow it and you'll not only reduce the causes of chronic inflammation, but you'll lower your risk of heart disease, diabetes, and other inflammation-related diseases as well.

EASING INFLAMMATION

The Doctor's Diet focuses on five ways to cool chronic inflammation.

1. LOWERING YOUR WEIGHT.

Excess weight sends out a red-alarm inflammatory alert in your body, and losing weight can help cool things down. Research shows that dropping even a small number of pounds can make a dramatic difference in inflammation levels.

In a 2012 study of overweight and obese women, researchers discovered that those who lost at least 5 percent of their body weight saw significant reductions in inflammation. After one year, those who lost weight through diet and exercise had a 41.7 percent reduction in C-reactive protein and a 24.3 percent cut in interleukin-6, two inflammatory markers that can be measured with blood tests. The study was published in the journal *Cancer Research*.

As you lose weight, your body's inflammation levels should start going down.

2. REDUCING EXPOSURE TO PRO-INFLAMMATORY FOODS.

Certain foods spark an inflammatory response, so it's best to avoid them or scale back on them. You'll find them in very limited amounts in The Doctor's Diet. They include:

✚ Highly processed carbohydrates—especially "white" foods such as white bread, sugary cereals, flour tortillas, and white rice

✚ Sugar-sweetened beverages, such as sodas, sweetened iced tea, fruit punches, and sports drinks

✚ Fast food, junk food, and deep-fried food

✚ Foods that contain trans fats (shortening, partially hydrogenated oils, most margarines, commercially made cakes and pastries)

MEASURING CHRONIC INFLAMMATION

Your doctor can order blood tests that look for certain inflammatory markers, such as C-reactive protein (CRP). The American Heart Association sets these guidelines for C-reactive protein levels in the blood:

✚ Less than 1 mg/dL: low risk
✚ 1 to 3 mg/dL: moderate risk
✚ 3 mg/dL or greater: high risk

People whose C-reactive protein levels are in the high-risk category have roughly twice the risk of heart attack compared to those in the low-risk group.

---

3. INCREASING YOUR EXPOSURE TO FOODS THAT COOL INFLAMMATION.

A variety of super-healthy foods help lower inflammation. That's why I've made them a major part of the Doctor's Diet. Most of the recommendations in my Food Prescriptions lower inflammation—that's one of the reasons I love these foods so much:

✚ Vegetables, especially those that are dark green, red, orange, and yellow. Like fruits, vegetables are a great source of phytochemicals, which are antioxidants that help your body in more ways than food scientists can count.

✚ Fruits, especially berries, which are relatively low in sugar and very high in antioxidants.

- High-fiber foods, such as whole grains (oats, quinoa, whole-grain breads) and legumes

- Nuts, such as walnuts, pecans, almonds, and peanuts

- Seeds, such as sesame seeds and flaxseeds

- Healthy fats in plant foods, such as olives and avocados

- Fatty fish, such as salmon, trout, herring, and tuna

- Vegetable and fruit oils, such as olive, canola, and safflower

- Herbs and spices, such as turmeric, ginger, garlic, basil, and pepper

---

Q: DOES CHOCOLATE REDUCE INFLAMMATION?

A: Studies show that cocoa in dark chocolate has the ability to slow the inflammation process. The flavonols in chocolate may also help lower LDL cholesterol, lower blood pressure, and improve insulin resistance. To maximize chocolate's health benefits without lots of extra calories, sugar, and fat, skip the milk chocolate and nibble on small amounts of dark chocolate that's at least 70 percent cocoa.

---

4. HELPING YOU LOSE BELLY FAT.

Having too much belly fat really turns on the burn when it comes to inflammation. Belly fat produces molecules called pro-inflammatory cytokines, which are molecules that trigger inflammation. Belly fat causes so much inflammation that it has been referred to as the "hotbed of inflammation."

As you improve your diet, lose weight, and add more activity into your daily life, you'll naturally whittle away belly fat and with it, your chronic, systemic inflammation.

5. EMPHASIZING THE HEALTH BENEFITS OF SLEEP.

I love making this recommendation. It's like telling people to eat more candy. Who doesn't love sleep?

Here's why I'm suggesting it: Poor sleep actually revs up chronic inflammation. When you don't get the sleep you need—either because you're staying up too late and getting up too early, or you have a sleep disorder that interferes with the quality of your sleep—inflammation increases as your body boosts its production of inflammatory chemicals.

In a 2010 study, Emory University researchers compared inflammation markers in people who slept fewer than six hours a night with those who slept six to nine hours. They found that those who got the least amount of shut-eye had higher levels of three inflammatory markers. For example, C-reactive protein levels were an average of 25 percent higher in the six-hour-per-night group.

Aim to get around seven to eight hours of sleep each night. Research shows that people who live the longest get about that much sleep, and they're less likely to be overweight along the way.

RESEARCH SHOWS THAT DROPPING EVEN A SMALL NUMBER OF POUNDS CAN MAKE A DRAMATIC DIFFERENCE IN INFLAMMATION LEVELS.

GETTING YOUR ZZZs

So now you know what inflammation is, why it matters, how to cool it down, and the many ways in which The Doctor's Diet can help fight it. You notice I mentioned that getting enough sleep is a natural anti-inflammatory. As it turns out, sleep has lots of other links to weight loss. Amazingly, the connections go both ways: not only does sleep help with weight loss, but weight loss can improve sleep. I'll tell you more about that next.

When it comes to sleep and weight, you're looking at a double-edged sword. Consistently getting too little sleep can raise your chances of gaining excess weight and becoming obese. That's one side of the sword. The other side is that gaining excess weight and becoming obese raise your chances of getting too little sleep.

So, as you can see, sleep and weight are connected in a continuous spiral that feeds upon itself. Sleeplessness leads to weight gain; weight gain leads to sleeplessness. How do you break free from this endless cycle?

In order to get truly healthy, you've got to work on both of these problems. Lose weight, and your sleep should improve. Get more sleep, and weight loss should be easier.

You're moving in the right direction by following The Doctor's Diet. You can take a few other steps as well, which I'll explain in this chapter. By making smart sleep choices, you'll be resting better in no time.

EASY BREATHING

Being overweight or obese affects sleep in several ways.

Excess weight can make it harder to breathe. As people gain weight, especially if fat collects in the neck and trunk area, breathing can become disordered. Fat can actually obstruct your airways, compromising respiratory function and interfering with your body's ability to get the oxygen it needs.

Problems with nighttime breathing can lead to a condition called sleep apnea, in which breathing pauses for short periods of time because airways become blocked. Sleep apnea can prevent people from sleeping deeply and from moving into all of the normal sleep phases their body needs to maintain good health. It is a leading cause of daytime sleepiness and is linked to other health problems, such as high blood pressure, heart attack, heart failure, stroke, diabetes, abnormal glucose metabolism, cognitive dysfunction, and driving accidents.

Sleep apnea can cause daytime sleepiness because you don't get the rest you really need, even if you spend the right number of hours in bed.

Having excess fat can interfere with sleep on a hormonal level as well. Fat cells, especially those in the belly, can produce abnormal levels of certain hormones that disrupt healthy sleep. When your sleep hormones are out of balance, it's harder to get the shut-eye you need.

WHAT IS SLEEP APNEA?

Sleep apnea is a common disorder in which people experience pauses in their breathing while they sleep. Breathing pauses can occur as many as 30 times an hour and can last from a few seconds to several minutes. Pauses may be followed by a snore, snort, or choking sound.

As many as 18 million Americans have sleep apnea; at least half are overweight or obese. As the obesity epidemic continues to grow, researchers are finding big spikes in the number of sleep apnea cases. In the past two decades, the number of people with sleep apnea has risen as much as 55 percent. The rise in American body weight is probably behind that increase, with 80 to 90 percent of the increased symptoms due to the rise in obesity.

One way sleep apnea is treated is with something called a nasal continuous positive airway pressure (CPAP) machine, which helps sufferers get the oxygen they need by keeping airways open during sleep.

Losing weight can also make a difference for people with sleep apnea. Reducing body weight by as little as 10 percent can lead to significant improvement of the disorder.

Sleep apnea often goes undiagnosed because people don't realize they are waking up during the night. But often they exhibit some of the signs of sleep apnea:

➕ Loud, frequent snoring, especially while on their back, and often noticed only by sleeping partners

➕ Choking or gasping for breath during sleep

- Daytime sleepiness

- Morning headaches, sore throat, or mouth dryness

- Problems with memory or learning

- Unexplained mood swings or personality changes

- Frequent nighttime awakenings, either to urinate or for no apparent reason

GREAT SLEEP FUELS WEIGHT LOSS

When you get enough sleep, weight loss becomes easier. Here are some of the reasons why:

- **You're revved to move.** It's easier to be active when you're well rested. Who wants to go out for a walk, a swim, or a jog when they can barely keep their eyes open?

- **Your metabolism is fully charged.** In studies where researchers have purposely disrupted the sleep of study participants, they find that after even just a few days, metabolism slows down. Getting enough sleep helps prevent that.

- **Your appetite hormones work better.** Being exhausted tends to increase your appetite and your calorie intake. That's because lack of sleep impacts your body's levels of leptin and ghrelin, hormones that are involved in hunger and satiety. (Ghrelin increases appetite, and leptin tells your body when to stop eating.) When your leptin and ghrelin levels are out of whack, you're much more likely to overeat, because your out-of-balance hormones are sending you false signals about hunger and satiety. Sleep helps keep them all in balance.

✚ **You have less time to overeat.** When people spend more time in bed, research shows that one of the things they spend less time doing is eating. The more awake time you have on your hands, the more you are likely to snack.

✚ **You're less likely to get mixed signals.** Tired people may eat more simply because they confuse feelings of fatigue and hunger. Instead of taking a nap when they feel tired, they gobble up food because they mistake that uncomfortable feeling of exhaustion for hunger.

✚ **It's easier to make healthy choices.** Well-rested people tend to make healthier decisions about what foods to eat. Given the choice of French fries or a salad, you're more likely to pick the fries if you're exhausted and the salad if you're well rested.

GETTING BETTER SLEEP

I'm happy to tell you that just as lack of sleep and weight gain are connected, so are better sleep and weight loss. Once you start eating right, being active, and losing weight, your sleep should begin to improve. And as it does, you should find it easier to eat right, be active, and lose weight. It's the vicious sleep-weight cycle in reverse.

Some other ways to improve sleep include making sure your sleep hygiene is up to snuff—that means making sure your bed, bedroom, and schedule are optimized for good sleep. And be sure to leave yourself enough time at night to relax and fall asleep and to get the seven to nine hours you need. You can't get eight hours of sleep if you're only in bed for six hours!

Q: HOW MUCH SLEEP DO I REALLY NEED?

A: Individual sleep needs vary, but in general, most of us do best with seven to nine hours of sleep.

TIPS FOR BETTER SLEEP

✚ Go to bed at the same time each night.

✚ Get up at the same time each morning.

✚ Be sure your bedroom is quiet, dark, and relaxing.

✚ Use earplugs, eye shades, light-blocking window shades, white noise machines, or whatever other tools you need to facilitate good sleep.

✚ Use heaters or air conditioners to make sure the temperature is right for sleeping.

✚ Sleep in a comfortable bed.

✚ Use your bed only for sleeping and having sex (doesn't sound too bad does it!).

✚ Remove all electronic entertainment devices from your bedroom. Don't watch TV, listen to music, talk on the phone, read on a tablet, use the computer, work, or do any other activities in bed.

✚ Avoid eating large meals before bed.

✚ Avoid exercising and doing other stimulating activities within a few hours before bed.

- Watch caffeine intake during the day; some people are so sensitive to it that a cup of coffee at lunchtime can affect their sleep.

- Keep in mind that caffeine sensitivity can change as you get older.

- If you're having trouble sleeping, or if your sleeping partner tells you that you're snoring, start keeping a sleep journal and discuss your findings with your doctor, who may refer you to a sleep center for further evaluation.

WELL-RESTED NURSES

The Nurses' Health Study, a large, long-term study conducted by the Harvard School of Public Health, followed roughly 60,000 women for 16 years, asking them about their weight, sleep habits, and other aspects of their lifestyle. Researchers found that women who slept five hours or less per night had a 15 percent higher risk of becoming obese, compared with women who slept seven hours per night.

REST EASY

Sleep energizes you—getting enough of it can really rev you up for a great day. Weight loss energizes you also. Once you start to really take control of your diet and your health, you'll probably find yourself smiling more than you used to. And once you start shedding excess pounds, you're likely to feel lighter emotionally as well as physically. Stay with me, and I'll tell you about another wonderful weight-loss payoff: high-octane energy that will help lift your mood.

We all know what it's like to be in a bad mood. Everything just seems kind of grey and dull. You may feel sad or lethargic, bored with activities that you usually enjoy, irritable with the people you come in contact with, discouraged and kind of hopeless that things are going to get better anytime soon. When these feelings last for a while, doctors diagnose depression, but for most of us, a blue mood is just something that comes and goes every now and then.

It's impossible—and unrealistic to expect—to be in a sunny mood all the time. But you can take steps to push your mood up a notch. In fact, one of the most enjoyable payoffs of following The Doctor's Diet is an improvement in your overall outlook on life.

Moodiness has many causes, from genetics to upbringing. But the choices you make every day about food and activity influence your mood as well. As with so many other aspects of health, the decisions you make throughout the day really do matter. By picking mood-boosting foods and eating patterns, losing weight, and zipping up your daily activity, you can optimize your emotional health, boost your mood, and energize your spirit.

WEIGHT LOSS: THE NATURAL MOOD ELEVATOR

Once you start following The Doctor's Diet and losing weight, you'll discover that releasing those excess pounds is one of the best mood boosters of all. Research bears this out: in studies with depressed people, those who lost weight reported feeling less depressed than those who didn't.

Part of that good feeling comes from obvious changes that accompany weight loss—of course you're going to feel better when your clothes aren't as snug, you have more energy, and you know you're making progress in your journey to better health. But there seems to be more to it than that. When you lose weight, the production of certain mood-impacting hormones can change. For example, losing weight can lead to lower levels of the stress hormone cortisol in your blood. Losing weight can also improve your body's ability to use the hormone insulin, which can help keep blood sugar—and mood—more stable.

When you start to see your weight go down, focus on how great it makes you feel. Congratulate yourself, and reinforce those good feelings. Even if your weight loss isn't happening as quickly as you might like, try to really enjoy the feeling of success. You might even want to spend a few minutes closing your eyes and visualizing all of the wonderful changes going on in your body as you lose weight. And give yourself credit for all of the healthy choices you're making! Small steps like these—acknowledging your hard work and really taking time to notice the benefits—not only lift your mood but help you stay on track.

START WITH YOUR PLATE

Food can affect your mood in a few ways. Certain foods contain substances or nutrients that actually contribute to mood improvement, so it's good to include those foods in your diet, as The Doctor's Diet does. Other kinds of food can impede your mood, so it's best to avoid them.

Let's start with the foods that support good mood:

FOODS THAT CONTAIN TRYPTOPHAN

Tryptophan is an essential amino acid, meaning your body needs it but cannot manufacture it (as it can with some other amino acids) so it must come from your diet. One of the ways your body uses tryptophan is to make serotonin, a brain chemical that helps regulate sleep and stabilize your mood. Serotonin is the brain chemical that is targeted by selective serotonin reuptake inhibitors (SSRIs), a class of antidepressant drug that includes fluoxetine (Prozac) and paroxetine (Paxil). Low levels of serotonin are associated with depression and anxiety.

Turkey is probably the best-known high-tryptophan food. Others include cheese, chicken, eggs, fish, milk, nuts, peanuts and peanut butter, pumpkin seeds, sesame seeds, soy, and tofu.

NUTS

There's a lot to love about the nutrients in nuts—which is why eating nuts is one of my most important Food Prescriptions. In terms of mood, the magnesium in nuts is important. Being low on magnesium can interfere with sleep, and as you know, it's hard to be in a great mood when you're sleep-deprived and exhausted.

Almonds, cashews, peanuts, and peanut butter provide good amounts of magnesium. Some other high-magnesium foods include wheat bran, spinach, raisin bran cereal, soybeans, wheat germ, oatmeal, and legumes. Brazil nuts are high in selenium, a nutrient that has also been associated with improved mood.

DARK CHOCOLATE

The cocoa in chocolate also helps boost blood levels of mood-improving serotonin. And compounds called polyphenols in chocolate help promote calmness and contentedness. Remember to go dark: the darker the chocolate, the more cocoa and less sugar it contains. Look for chocolate with a high percentage of cocoa (ideally over 70 percent), because cocoa is the source of chocolate's health benefits. And limit yourself to a small piece (about half an ounce) per serving because the calories can add up.

I do want to add a caveat to this advice, though: some people can eat a small piece of dark chocolate and stop there. But for others—you know who you are—all it does is set off a craving, and before you know it you're gobbling up candy bars. If eating dark chocolate just triggers your chocoholicism, skip it—there are plenty of other mood-boosters that won't end up costing you hundreds of empty calories.

WHOLE GRAINS

Keeping blood sugar at a stable level throughout the day helps keep your mood even because when blood sugar falls, so does your mood. One way to keep blood sugar at an even keel is to avoid getting too hungry. You can do this by eating a meal or snack every three to four hours. Make sure those meals and snacks contain the right combination of protein, healthy fats, and whole grains, because too much of one and too little of another can make blood sugar go up and down.

Whole grains help your mood in another way as well. Complex carbohydrates contribute to your brain's manufacturing of serotonin. And they tend to be good sources of folate, a B vitamin. Research has found that depressed people may have lower blood folate levels than those who are not depressed, so it makes sense to keep an eye on your folate intake.

FOODS WITH OMEGA-3 FATTY ACIDS

When I eat foods that contain omega-3 fatty acids, I feel as if my mood zips up just thinking about how great they are for my health. As we discussed earlier, omega-3s bring a lot to the table in terms of health benefits: they reduce inflammation and help your heart, your brain, and your joints in a variety of ways. They can also help raise your mood—in fact, studies suggest they may help reduce depressive symptoms in people with clinical depression.

Top sources of omega-3 fatty acids include flax seeds, walnuts, sardines, salmon, mackerel, herring, soybeans, tofu, and shrimp.

FOODS WITH VITAMIN D

Levels of vitamin D are sometimes low in depressed people, and some small studies have found connections between vitamin D and mood. While the researchers figure out the details, go ahead and keep your vitamin D levels up, because it's great for bone health, lowers inflammation, aids your immune system, and may help ward off some kinds of cancer.

Top sources of vitamin D include salmon, tuna, and vitamin D–enriched milk, orange juice, and breakfast cereals.

Failing to get enough iron can lead to fatigue, moodiness, lack of focus, and an overall feeling of having very little energy in your tank.

Top sources of iron include red meat, oysters, spinach, legumes, dried fruit, turkey, tuna, egg yolks, and iron-fortified cereals.

WANT TO BE HAPPY? HAVE HAPPY FRIENDS

We know that social support—having friends and family that love us, support us, listen to us, and enjoy being with us—adds to our psychological happiness. But studies have also found that spending time with happy people makes us happier, and being with negative, critical people can bring us down. Likewise, surrounding ourselves with people who eat a healthy diet, exercise, and try to maintain a healthy weight can rub off on us in a positive way.

As you make life-saving changes to your diet and as you strive to add more activity to your days, try to socialize with like-minded people and limit your contact with those who disrespect your goals or criticize your intentions. When it comes to your health, positive attitudes and wise choices can be contagious.

Now is a great time to branch out and form new friendships. Reach out to others who share your new health goals and make them a part of your life. By building a supportive community of health-focused friends, neighbors, and family, you'll have plenty of people standing beside you to help you as you face challenges and to cheer with you as you celebrate milestones.

Just as there are foods that boost mood, there are foods that can bring your mood down.

Start with processed foods made with refined carbohydrates, low-quality fats, salt, sugar, artificial flavors, food additives, hydrogenated fats, and all kinds of chemicals. These are not the foods our bodies were designed to use as fuel, and eating them is like putting trash in your car's gas tank instead of gasoline. Simple carbohydrates and sugar cause blood sugar spikes and falls that send your mood up and down like a ping-pong ball. Cheap, low-quality oils put a strain on your system as it fights to digest these highly processed, toxin-filled fats. And who knows what our bodies are thinking when they try to handle all the additives in these pseudo-foods.

Eating junk food can push your mood up temporarily. If we think of them as treats, our brains react by saying, "Yay! Cupcakes!" or "Yum! Potato chips!" We've been conditioned to get excited by these "special" foods. But once we start really paying attention to how they make us feel, we realize that the good feeling doesn't last long.

Start paying attention to how these foods make you feel. You might be surprised by how much they impact your mood. A friend of mine got into a habit of buying a candy bar when she would stop at the grocery store for dinner supplies. She'd be hungry after a long day at work, and she'd "treat" herself to a candy bar, thinking it would give her the energy she needed to haul the groceries home and get a healthy dinner on the table.

When she really started to pay attention to how certain foods made her feel, though, she noticed that while getting dinner ready she often felt sick to her stomach. She also realized she was short-tempered with her kids. She assumed both of these feelings were caused by the stress of the evening rush, but then she started to wonder if the candy bar had anything to do with it. One day she skipped the candy bar and grabbed a bottle of veggie juice instead. She was amazed at how much better she felt—no icky stomach, and, even better, she wasn't snapping at her kids. Once she noticed this, she started paying attention to how other foods made her feel, and it became obvious that eating junk food made her mood suffer. Realizing this made it much easier for her to make smarter choices. Sure, junk food may taste good going down, but if it leaves you feeling cranky, sad, exhausted, and unmotivated, it's just not worth eating.

As for eating junk in an effort to get yourself out of a bad mood, don't bother, because it really doesn't work. Research has found that when people who are concerned with their weight and their diet binge on junk food, their moods get even worse—no surprise there.

ONE OF THE BEST MOOD RAISERS OF ALL

There's no two ways about it: getting out there and moving your body is a major mood booster. Study after study has found strong links between exercise and mood. In a nutshell, the findings show that active people are less likely to become depressed than inactive people, and active people who stop exercising are more likely to get depressed than people who stay active. Research even shows that for some people with major depression, exercise is as effective a treatment as antidepressant medication.

And here's the best part: activity can have an almost immediate impact on your mood. Psychology researchers say that mood can begin to improve just five minutes after you start exercising moderately. Five minutes! There aren't many other health interventions that start to work that quickly.

For these reasons—and so many others—I truly hope you're making activity a part of your daily life.

Exercise's mood-raising effects seem to come from changes in serotonin, dopamine, and other feel-good brain chemicals that activate when you exercise. An enjoyable workout—whether it's swimming laps in a pool, walking around your neighborhood, jogging on the high school track, taking a Zumba class with friends—also gives you a great sense of accomplishment that lingers for hours. Our psyches feel pleased when we engage in a meaningful activity, so exercise can make you feel as good about yourself as doing volunteer work. It also lowers the levels of stress hormones such as cortisol in your blood.

A good mood is sort of like money: no matter how much you have, it's always nice to have more. Whether or not you struggle with feelings of sadness, depression, or anxiety, following The Doctor's Diet should help improve your mood. It starts with good eating: when you focus on the whole, healthful foods that make up The Doctor's Diet eating plan, you're filling your plate with mood-boosting foods and staying away from foods that bring you down. When you exercise, you enjoy psychological and physiological benefits that can start to cheer you up within minutes and last for hours. And when you start shedding pounds, you'll feel fantastic about yourself, not only because you'll look better but because you'll be setting the stage for a longer, healthier, happier life. Those are some great reasons to feel good about yourself!

And here's another reason to feel great: losing weight can lower your risk of a disease that we all fear. Stay tuned and I'll tell you more about that.

> "OBESITY IS A MAJOR RISK FACTOR FOR DEVELOPING CANCER, ROUGHLY THE EQUIVALENT OF TOBACCO USE, AND BOTH ARE POTENTIALLY REVERSIBLE. FURTHER, OBESE CANCER PATIENTS DO WORSE IN SURGERY, WITH RADIATION, OR ON CHEMOTHERAPY—WORSE BY ANY MEASURE."
> —KAREN BASEN-ENGQUIST, PhD, UNIVERSITY OF TEXAS MD ANDERSON CANCER CENTER

The statistics truly are staggering. In 2013, doctors diagnosed 1.6 million new cases of cancer, and 580,350 Americans died from the disease. And here's the part that really hurts: one-quarter to one-third of those cancers were caused by poor nutrition, physical inactivity, and excess weight. That's right. Nearly 200,000 of those deaths could have been prevented—not by miracle drugs or amazing cures, but by the very same lifestyle choices that you're making as part of The Doctor's Diet.

Cancer is a complicated disease—in fact, there are actually hundreds of diseases that fit under the wide label of "cancer." It's really only recently that researchers have started to tease out the connections between diet, weight, and cancer. But despite the fact that there are still so many unanswered questions, one fact stands out: excess weight fuels cancer risk.

How sure are we of this? Let me share with you a quote on the topic that jumped out at me when I first read it. Scientific researchers are not big on absolutes—they're much more likely to err on the side of caution and say certain things "might" cause disease rather than saying they "do" cause disease. But when it comes to weight and cancer, there's no beating around the bush by W. Philip T. James, MD, a member of the panel of World Cancer Research Fund experts who analyzed 7,000 studies of weight and cancer:

"The message is absolutely clear as a bell: the relation of cancer to obesity is so robust, it is going to rank close to the smoking problem in America pretty soon."

OK, so we've established that excess weight boosts cancer risk. Now let's talk about why that connection exists—and how following The Doctor's Diet may lower your chances of getting it.

CANCERS LINKED WITH WEIGHT

Excess weight is associated with an increased risk of certain cancers, including cancers of the:

✚ Esophagus
✚ Breast (postmenopausal)
✚ Endometrium (lining of the uterus)
✚ Colon and rectum
✚ Kidney
✚ Pancreas
✚ Thyroid
✚ Gallbladder
✚ Liver
✚ Cervix
✚ Ovary
✚ Blood (non-Hodgkin's lymphoma and multiple myeloma)
✚ Prostate (aggressive forms)

Aside from weight, inactivity is associated with an increased risk of these cancers of the:

✚ Colon
✚ Breast
✚ Endometrium
✚ Lung

In addition, excess weight is associated with worse outcomes among some cancer patients, particularly those with cancer of the breast, prostate, and colon.

Our bodies are made up of trillions of cells that are constantly growing and dividing. Sometimes—because of genetic mutations, environmental damage, or other reasons—cells can begin to grow and spread abnormally. When this growth is not stopped or controlled, cancer develops.

Some people are way more apt to get cancer than others. Smokers, for example, have a very high risk of getting lung cancer because cigarette smoke contains at least 69 known carcinogens.

In animal studies, scientists see that compared with normal-weight animals, tumors in fat animals grow faster and larger, spread more quickly, and are more resistant to treatment. Observational studies find similar trends in people: overweight and obese people get more cancer, their cancer gets worse, and they are more likely to die from it than people of normal weight.

Why is this? Why are people who are overweight or obese more likely to get cancer than those whose weight is normal? Here are some of the reasons:

✦ **Extra weight equals extra estrogen.** Body fat produces estrogen, and estrogen fuels some kinds of cancer, such as estrogen-positive breast cancer and endometrial cancer. The more fat you have, the more estrogen you have in your blood.

✦ **Insulin resistance sets the stage for cancer development and tumor growth.** Overweight and obese people are likely to have insulin resistance, which we talked about back in the section on blood sugar. If you are insulin resistant, your blood is likely to have high levels of insulin and a substance called insulin-like growth factor-1 (IGF-1). Both insulin and IGF-1 seem to promote the growth of certain kinds of tumors because they help regulate cell division.

✦ **Fat cells produce cancer-spurring proteins.** Your body's fat cells— especially the fat cells that take up residence in your belly—release proteins known as adipokines, which can play a part in cell growth. People with excess belly fat tend to have lower levels of the protein adiponectin, which helps prevent the growth of cancer cells. And they are likely to have higher levels of leptin, which seems to promote the proliferation of cancer cells.

✚ **Fat may turn cancer genes "on."** Only about 5 percent of cancers are related to genetic mutations. But not everyone who has certain cancer-causing genetic mutations goes on to develop cancer. Scientists believe certain factors (such as environmental toxins, diet, body fat, smoking, and others) may have the ability to "turn on" some cancer genes. It appears that having excess body fat seems to contribute to the turning on of genes linked to cancer in people with a genetic predisposition.

✚ **Excess weight boosts inflammation.** As we discussed earlier in the book, having extra body weight and body fat—especially belly fat—turns up the heat on chronic systemic inflammation, which appears to contribute to the development of some kinds of cancer.

✚ **Inactivity contributes, too.** People who are overweight or obese are less likely than healthy-weight folks to get enough exercise. Since exercise helps ward off cancer, inactivity is believed to be one of the links in the cancer-weight connection. Activity spurs the action of several cancer-fighting events: it lowers inflammation, boosts immunity, lowers levels of pro-cancer hormones such as estrogen in the blood, helps regulate leptin (known as the "weight hormone"), and improves blood sugar and insulin resistance.

✚ OBESE WOMEN HAVE A 62 PERCENT HIGHER RISK OF DYING FROM CANCER THAN WOMEN OF NORMAL WEIGHT; FOR OBESE MEN, THE DEATH RATE FROM CANCER IS 52 PERCENT HIGHER.

LOSING WEIGHT, LOWERING RISK

Cancer takes a long time to develop. As many as 10 years can go by before the early cellular changes of cancer cause signs and symptoms that can be detected by people and their doctors. So it's a little hard for researchers to make surefire connections between weight loss and reduction of cancer risk. However, there is a fair amount of evidence that making changes like the ones in The Doctor's Diet can bring down cancer risk.

For example, a large 2006 study published in the *Journal of the American Medical Association* found that women who lost 4 to 11 pounds after menopause had a more than 20 percent lower risk of breast cancer compared to women whose weight did not change. Not all studies have shown this same benefit, but heck, it's evidence enough for me to encourage all the women I know to try to lose extra pounds.

Studies also suggest that increased activity may help prevent cancer of the colon, breast, prostate, lung, and endometrium. For example, some research has shown that physical activity can reduce risk of endometrial cancer by 20 to 40 percent and lung cancer by 20 percent. In my book, those are odds worth shooting for.

Making changes like those in The Doctor's Diet can help cancer survivors as well as those who have never had cancer. Research has found that breast cancer survivors who exercise moderately (three to five hours per week at an average pace) have better survival rates than those who don't. Other studies show that colon cancer is less likely to recur in people who exercise.

The bottom line? By following the recommendations in The Doctor's Diet—eating a healthy diet, losing weight, shedding belly fat, becoming more active—you can take significant steps toward lowering your risk of many kinds of cancer. And if you've already started following my plan, congratulations—you're already on your way to lowering your cancer risk!

MOVING TO PREVENT COLON CANCER

Many studies have looked at the connection between colon cancer and exercise. Overall they've found that adults who increase their physical activity, either by exercising harder, longer, or more frequently, can lower their chance of developing colon cancer by 30 to 40 percent compared with sedentary people. The benefit is especially strong in people who do 30 to 60 minutes a day of moderate to vigorous physical activity.

WEIGHT AND BREAST CANCER

Many studies have found a connection between excess weight and postmenopausal breast cancer—especially for tumors whose growth is fueled by the hormones estrogen and progesterone. Postmenopausal women who are overweight or obese have a 30 to 60 percent higher breast cancer risk than those who are at a healthy body weight.

Fat tissue contains an enzyme called aromatase that converts hormones (androgens) into estrogen. So it's not surprising that having excess body fat raises the amount of estrogen in the blood—and with it, the risk of estrogen-positive breast cancer.

TELL YOUR DAUGHTERS: GET MOVING!

Studies suggest that vigorous physical activity during adolescence can offer strong protection against breast cancer later in life. If you have a teen daughter, encourage her to walk, run, cycle, swim, join sports teams, and be as active as possible.

ONE MORE PAYOFF

We've covered a lot of ground here. We've looked at the many physical and emotional payoffs that come with weight loss. But I don't want to stop here. You may not realize it, but when you make life-changing choices in your diet and activity levels and drop excess weight, the payoffs go beyond you. Following The Doctor's Diet and living a truly healthy life pays off for your family as well as yourself. And believe it or not, it even impacts family members that haven't even been born yet!

Stay tuned, and I'll tell you more about one of the best weight-loss payoffs of all: a healthier family.

As you follow The Doctor's Diet and start to lose weight, renew your health, cut your risk of disease, and pump up your chances of living a longer, more vibrant life, you're not just giving yourself the gift of health—you're doing something amazing for your family, too. Taking charge of your diet, weight, and commitment to being active can positively impact your family's health now and for years—even generations—to come.

I know that sounds dramatic, but it really is true. As researchers analyze the causes and effects of America's obesity epidemic, they're learning that the choices we make now truly can affect our family for a very long time.

Here's an example. Being overweight or obese during pregnancy makes it much more likely that you'll have a large-birthweight baby. Big babies make for a more complicated pregnancy—they're harder to deliver, so their moms are more likely to need Cesarean sections, which are riskier than ordinary vaginal births. Big babies also tend to have more health issues during and after birth.

But the potential problems don't end there. Large birthweight babies tend to grow into overweight toddlers, children, teens, and adults. It's true—big babies are more likely than normal-weight babies to be overweight or obese for their entire lives. So a mom who gains too much weight while she's pregnant is setting her child up for a lifetime of weight-related struggles.

Sure, there are some genetic and social factors at play. But those don't explain everything. When a fetus is growing inside its mother, Mom's excess weight actually seems to affect the fetus in a physiological, biochemical way. The fetus seems to receive some kind of cellular or hormonal imprints that predisposes it to a lifetime of extra weight.

I'm not saying this to make anyone feel guilty. I know it's the kind of thing that can be hard to hear, especially if you're an overweight or obese woman who's given birth to a large baby. I'm saying it to drive home an important point about being overweight: it affects the people around you, often in a negative way. Fortunately the flip side is true as well: losing weight and restoring good health also affects the people around you—but it does so in a positive, life-saving way. You have power to impact your own destiny and your family's destiny as well.

It's never too late to choose life and health, both for yourself and for your family. That's one of the things that excite me most about The Doctor's Diet: by using it to design a new way of life for yourself, you're also taking major steps to build a stronger, healthier family. The changes you make today could echo through the lives of the people you love for years to come.

By following The Doctor's Diet, making smart changes in your diet, exercise, and weight, you're setting an amazing example for your spouse, children, parents, relatives, neighbors, friends, co-workers—even the guy behind the counter at your local coffee shop, where you've switched from a daily donut and an iced latte to a coffee with a little milk.

Every time you choose a glass of seltzer over a soda, every time you toss a scrumptious salad instead of ordering a pizza, every time you go for a walk with a pal instead of plopping down on the couch with a massive bowl of potato chips, you're modeling healthy behavior for the people around you. You're showing them that healthy choices are possible and enjoyable.

Even dogs benefit when their owners get smart about diet and exercise. As many as half of all pets are overweight or obese, and if you bring your dog along on your walks, he'll see many of the same health benefits as you. (Sorry, The Doctor's Diet probably won't work for cats, unless you have one of those rare felines who enjoys walking on a leash!)

Listen, we're all looking for inspiration and motivation. That's what you can give the people in your life when you start living a healthier life. Your enthusiasm and commitment can rub off on them, whether they're adults or kids. It may not happen right away, or with everyone in your life, but I'm telling you—people will be watching you, and they'll be guided by your smart choices.

Being a model of healthy behavior is just one way to spread the news about your new life-saving approach to diet and exercise. You can also take a more direct route, by working with the people you love to make changes in their lives.

Here are some ideas on how to do this. Remember, not every idea will work in your house—people have different ways of approaching healthy change, and sometimes if you're too heavy-handed, your advice backfires. (Got teenagers? Then you know what I mean.) So before you implement any big shifts in how you run your house, make sure you're taking the approach that's best for your family. Some of these tips work best for younger children; others come in handy if the people in your family circle are older.

WE'RE ALL LOOKING FOR INSPIRATION AND MOTIVATION. THAT'S WHAT YOU CAN GIVE THE PEOPLE IN YOUR LIFE WHEN YOU START LIVING A HEALTHIER LIFE.

TALK IT UP

The way you explain your new way of eating can have a big effect on how people perceive it. If you moan and groan about how hard it is and how much you're giving up, nobody's going to want to follow your lead. But if you focus on the positive, sharing your excitement and emphasizing all the health benefits and surprisingly tasty combinations of your new eating plan, people's interest will be piqued, and they'll be more likely to want to give it a try, too.

That's not to say that you've got to make it seem like changing your diet is nothing but sunshine and happiness. I know there are going to be some challenges with change, and commiserating with others can be a helpful way to face them. But if your goal is to help your family adopt your new way of life, a positive, optimistic attitude will go a lot further than an earful of grumbling.

SHOP TOGETHER

The grocery store is a great place to think about healthy, nutritious food. Instead of just walking down the aisles tossing foods into your cart, take time to talk with family members about what you're buying. You don't want to spend the whole trip lecturing about the health benefits of spinach, but maybe you can steer them in the direction of a new fruit or veggie. Maybe if they help pick out the ingredients for a stir-fry, they'll be more interested in eating it. Maybe they'll learn how to read a food label, and why it's important. So often we're on autopilot in the grocery store, buying the same things over and over. But when you slow down and look around, you can make healthier choices—and so can the people you shop with.

COOK TOGETHER

Preparing a meal with other people can be an enjoyable experience, and it's also an opportunity to brainstorm about healthy ways to create tasty foods. Experiment with spices and herbs; look for ways to give new, healthy twists to dishes you've been making for years. While you're cooking, enjoy each other's company.

EAT TOGETHER

You've probably heard the research on this: families who sit down together for a healthy meal fare better than those who don't—not just in weight, but in social ways as well. Shut off the TV, sit down together, and enjoy a healthy meal with the people you love.

EXERCISE TOGETHER

This is a great way to spend time with friends and family. Instead of meeting for a heavy meal, grab your best buds and go for a walk or hike. You'll have plenty of quality time for talking and catching up. And you'll be amazed at how the miles fly by! Head for a park, a high school track, a ritzy part of town, a wooded path—even just a stroll through your own neighborhood is a great way to be active and enjoy time with pals.

If you have kids, invite them to walk with you—you may be surprised how often they say yes. This works even better if you have a dog. If there's no pooch in your house, offer to walk your neighbor's—I don't know any person or dog who would say no to that!

Many parents find that a walk in the evening is a nice time to connect with kids—especially teens. Kids have a lot on their minds these days, and sometimes when you're out walking, they start to talk. Things come up that may not when you're home—stories about friends, worries about school, their opinions about what's going on in their lives or the world. There's something about walking together that opens kids up. The process of walking relaxes them, and with no television, computers, or other people to compete with, they feel good having your attention.

SET A SMART-SNACKING EXAMPLE

Sitting down to watch a movie with your family? Hey, I'm not telling you not to snack. It's OK to have a little something while you're watching a flick. But when you haul out a giant bag of chips with a massive tub of unhealthy dip, you're setting a pretty bad example. Instead, set out some healthy snacks—vegetables and hummus, sliced fruit, or whole-grain crackers and guacamole, for example. Remember, the goal is to enjoy watching a movie together, not to have a giant load of unhealthy food while you're doing it.

WORK TOGETHER ON PORTION CONTROL

It's happened so slowly that you may not have noticed, but portion sizes in America have gotten bigger and bigger over the years. Muffins, donuts, sodas, hamburgers—everything is two or three times bigger now than it was a generation ago. Even the dishes are bigger: a friend of mine showed me a set of 1960s nested mixing bowls she inherited from her mother, and we both were amazed to see that the smallest bowl in the set—the one my friend remembered using to mix a banana bread recipe when she was a child—was the exact same size as the cereal bowl in a set of new dishes she had recently bought.

You may remember when portion sizes were smaller, but your kids probably don't. They may think 32 ounces is one serving of soda rather than four. Talk with them about this. Help them eat intelligent-sized portions. Show them that the bagel they are biting into is actually three servings rather than one. I'm not suggesting you be obnoxious about it— kids don't like being force-fed advice on how much to eat. But if you can find ways to share this information in a supportive way, you'll be doing them a real service.

Be honest with your kids. Hey, you enjoy a double-scoop ice cream cone as much as the next person. But help them to understand that it makes so much more sense to stick to healthy-sized portions. Most of the enjoyment of something like ice cream comes in the first few bites, anyway. It comes down to immediate gratification vs. long-term thinking. And let's face it: kids are terrible at delaying gratification about anything, not just food. Any parent who's watched a kid play video games instead of studying for their spelling test knows that. But your job as a parent is to help teach kids about the value of making smart choices that pay off over the long term.

RECONSIDER WHAT FOODS YOU BRING INTO YOUR HOUSE

This is something you have to think about carefully in relation to the personalities of the people you live with. Lots of nutrition experts tell you to do a full-scale clean-out of your kitchen and get rid of every speck of food that isn't on their approved lists. I agree with that to some extent—you're not going to inhale a gallon of chocolate ice cream if there's none in the freezer. But let's face it: if you have a house full of teenagers and you leave nothing for them to eat but quinoa and lentils, they're going to rebel. My advice is to get rid of as much of the junk as possible, but do so within the parameters of your own family's reality.

If you can't do a clean sweep, settle for a swap. If your family won't give up their ice cream, limit the amount you keep in the freezer. If they insist on having chips in the cabinet, pick the healthiest kind you can find. And remember that for some family members, a gradual approach with their eventual buy-in may end up being way more successful than renting an industrial-size trash bin and filling it with everyone's favorite foods while they're not looking.

AVOID FAST FOOD

I get it—after a long day, it's nice to be able to zip over to a fast-food joint and pick up a drive-thru dinner in minutes. But fast food is usually such an unhealthy choice, both for you and your family. Studies have found that people who frequent fast-food restaurants pay the price with excess weight.

A 2009 study published in the *Journal of Nutrition*, which followed

3,000 young adults for 13 years, discovered that people who had higher fast-food intake levels at the start of the study weighed an average of about 13 pounds more than people who had the lowest fast-food intake levels. They also had larger waist circumferences and greater increases in triglycerides. You may feel like you're saving time eating fast food, but considering that a lifetime of too many burgers and fries could contribute to a shorter life, regularly eating fast food doesn't seem like such a great idea.

PLAN ACTIVE VACATIONS

There are loads of ways to be active and still have an enjoyable, relaxing vacation. Instead of just lying on the beach for a week, choose trips with built-in active fun. Go cycling along boardwalks, hiking in national parks, swimming in lakes, and so on. All of my favorite vacations have been packed with activity and the memories they have created.

LIMIT SCREEN TIME

This is a big one. Studies have found that the more time adults and children spend in front of televisions and computers, the more likely they are to carry around excess weight. We all like our screen time, but all that sitting (and the snacking that usually goes along with it) adds up to weight gain. You can limit your kids' screen time by keeping televisions, computers, and phones out of their bedrooms. Limit yours by planning non-screen ways to relax. Instead of watching TV, head out for a walk or a bike ride. It's fine to veg out in front of the screen sometimes, but make it a treat, not a habit.

MAKE SURE YOUR KIDS GET ENOUGH SLEEP.

Children who don't get enough sleep are more likely to gain weight. A 2005 *British Medical Journal* study of 8,000 children found that those who slept fewer than 10.5 hours a night at age 3 had a 45 percent higher risk of becoming obese by age 7, compared with children who slept more than 12 hours nightly. A 2008 *Pediatrics* study found that each one-hour reduction in sleep during childhood was associated with a 50 percent higher risk of obesity at age 32.

The bottom line: set an example of good sleep for your children. Talk to them about the importance of sleep and its impact on health, and help them arrange their schedules to allow for enough sleep time. Keep computers, televisions, and phones out of the bedroom, and make sure your children's bedrooms are dark enough, quiet enough, and the right temperature for sleeping.

HAPPY AND FAT?

Does a good marriage lead to weight gain? Unfortunately, a 2013 study published in the journal *Health Psychology* found the answer to that question may be yes. Researchers discovered that young newlyweds who are satisfied with their marriage gained more weight than those who were less satisfied.

I would have expected the opposite, but the researchers' explanation makes sense. They believe that those who are satisfied are less motivated to attract an alternative mate. In other words, feeling secure with your spouse may lead you to relax your efforts to maintain your weight because you're not out trying to find someone to date.

This doesn't mean we should get divorced in order to stay lean. But I think it does suggest that when we think of weight just in terms of appearance, we're likely to lose focus when we feel we look good enough—or as we get older and we become more realistic about valuing other things over appearance. If we look at weight as being about health rather than vanity, we can work together with our mates to reach a healthy weight and have a satisfying relationship. In fact, I think that a common goal of eating right, being active, and aiming for a healthy weight can nurture a relationship in a positive way.

FACTS ABOUT KIDS AND WEIGHT

✚ Obesity rates have doubled in children and tripled in adolescents in the past three decades.

✚ Overall, about 33 percent of youths age 6 to 19 are overweight, and 18 percent are obese.

✚ Rates vary among ethnic groups: 26 percent of African American, 23 percent of Hispanic, and 15 percent of white youth are obese.

✚ Although genetic factors play a role in youth obesity, an overall change in calories consumed vs. calories burned during the past 30 years is believed to be the major cause of kids and teens becoming overweight or obese. Basically, kids today eat much more and exercise much less than earlier generations.

✚ Obese youth are likely to have high cholesterol, high blood pressure, high blood sugar, bone and joint problems, sleep apnea, poor self-esteem, and social problems.

✚ Overweight and obese kids are highly likely to grow up to be overweight or obese adults. Many of the health risks faced by obese adults are worse when they start in childhood—which is why it's so important to try to help overweight and obese kids lose weight through healthy eating and exercise.

There you have it—a list of weight-loss payoffs a mile long. You probably knew all along that weight loss was worth it, but now you really understand the many advantages of losing weight and choosing to live a healthier life!

It's time to move on to the next—and final—part of The Doctor's Diet: the MAINTAIN Plan. Starting the MAINTAIN Plan is a bit like graduating from school—you've worked really hard, won many victories, and learned a lot about yourself, and now it's time to begin the journey that will lead you through the rest of your life.

PART FIVE
THE DOCTOR'S DIET MAINTAIN PLAN

You've done it!

You've faced your weight emergency head-on and have made major changes in your diet.

You've shed your excess pounds, burned off life-threatening body fat, lowered disease risk, and taken many giant steps on the pathway toward a longer, healthier life.

You've completed the STAT Plan and the RESTORE Plan. Now you're ready to move on to a lifetime of good health with the MAINTAIN Plan.

The MAINTAIN Plan does just what its name implies: it helps you maintain all of the weight loss and health benefits that you worked so hard to achieve. However, because your goal is to maintain weight loss rather than shed pounds, the MAINTAIN Plan focuses a little less on cutting back and gives you a lot more leeway with your food choices.

I'm really excited to introduce you to the MAINTAIN Plan because it gives you the space to experiment a little more and have some fun with the healthy new foods you've discovered.

MAINTAIN IS A PLAN FOR LIFE

This is how I live my life. I don't think of it as a diet at all—I just think of it as how I eat every day! I *enjoy* my meals not only because they taste good, but because I know they're contributing to my good health. I don't stress out about counting calories (but I am very aware of my portion sizes). Sure, I make modifications here and there when I know my activity level is lower or higher, but it's not the least bit complicated. I think you'll also find this is surprisingly easy and a whole heck of a lot of fun.

The MAINTAIN Plan is designed around the secret to long-term weight-loss success: continuing to make smart choices about what you eat, keeping a close eye on portion sizes, and being as active as possible.

With the MAINTAIN Plan, there's no looking back. It's all about looking forward to having a slimmer, healthier body for the rest of your life. The best way to do that is to keep eating the foods that have brought you success so far.

The MAINTAIN Plan is a simple prescription for good health that will last you a lifetime. You can do this part of the The Doctor's Diet forever—for the rest of your long, healthy life. Sure, you may "slip up" now and then, but because this isn't one of those super-restrictive, unappetizing fad diets, you won't deviate nearly as much as you have on plans you've tried in the past. In fact, by now, I'm willing to bet that you're so in love with healthy foods and how they make you feel that you aren't even thinking about those less-healthy choices you used to make.

The MAINTAIN Plan is a culmination of all the great advice, tips, approaches, and information you've learned about so far. But it also builds in some extra freedom and flexibility that allow you to tailor it completely to your personal tastes. The MAINTAIN Plan is so customizable that you can truly make it your own.

The MAINTAIN Plan is built around eight winning strategies that pave the way for continued success. Follow these eight strategies and you'll maintain your weight loss forever. That sounds pretty great, doesn't it?

THE MAINTAIN MEAL PLAN EQUATIONS

I provide Meal Plan Equations for the MAINTAIN Plan because some people prefer to use them. It's up to you: you can follow these equations closely if that's what will work best for you, or just use them as guidelines, using the numbers on the scale to make adjustments over time. I want you to have as much structure or flexibility as you need—remember, this is about you eating a diet that will keep *you* and *your* weight healthy for the rest of *your* life.

MAINTAIN BREAKFAST:
  1 Breakfast Protein + 1 Fruit

MAINTAIN LUNCH:
  1 Main-Dish Protein + 2 or more Anytime Vegetables

MAINTAIN DINNER:
  1 Main-Dish Protein + 2 or more Anytime Vegetables

MAINTAIN SNACK #1:
  1 Snack Protein + 1 Fruit

MAINTAIN SNACK #2:
  1 Snack Protein + 1 or more Anytime Vegetables

DAILY FLEX-TIME FOODS:
  Each day enjoy these additional foods smartly based on your
  metabolism and activity levels:

+ Healthy Fats
+ Carb-Flex Foods:
  -Whole Grains
  -High-Density Vegetables
  -Anytime Vegetables
  -Fruits
+ Optional Alcohol-based Beverage (Max: 1 per day for women,
  2 per day for men)

MAINTAIN PLAN MEALS

Food lists on MAINTAIN are the same as STAT and RESTORE. And if you like a daily glass of wine or other Alcohol-based Beverages, there's room for it in the MAINTAIN Plan.

More than anything else, the MAINTAIN Plan is about *choice*.

The MAINTAIN Plan allows you to make your own choices about what to eat. Ultimately, I want YOU to fill in all the blanks and create healthy meals that you love and look forward to. There's so much flexibility in the MAINTAIN Plan that anyone who follows it will have a different daily menu. At this stage if you want to occasionally add in regular potatoes as a high-density vegetable, by all means do so, but just remember, regular potatoes can raise blood sugar quickly and should be eaten in moderation.

If you're someone who doesn't like all that flexibility and freedom, it's fine to stick with the RESTORE menus. Pick and choose your favorite foods. Just make sure you keep an eye on portion sizes and the types of foods you eat. In general, the key to the MAINTAIN plan is discovering the correct portion sizes of the healthy foods you enjoy that allow you to stay at your ideal body weight.

The STAT and RESTORE Plan gave you two weeks of daily menus. Because the MAINTAIN Plan is more flexible, I'm going to open things up a bit and list a variety of options for each meal. That gives you the freedom to choose what you like best—and to add your own creations as well.

BREAKFAST CHOICES

+ Smoothies made with fruit and milk or yogurt
+ Scrambled eggs or egg whites
+ Omelets made with vegetables
+ Yogurt mixed with fruit and nuts
+ Oatmeal
+ Whole-grain toast, or whole-grain English muffins spread with nut butter
+ Apples or pears spread with nut butter
+ Cottage cheese mixed with fruit

LUNCH CHOICES

+ Vegetable-based soups
+ Bean and lentil soups
+ Garden salads
+ Salads with fish, shellfish, or chicken

- Open-faced sandwiches on whole-grain bread made with lean meat, vegetables, nut butters, and/or avocado
- Baked fish, poultry, or lean meat with vegetables
- Bean-based dishes
- Chili

SNACK CHOICES

- Fruit
- Raw veggies dipped in hummus or guacamole
- Nuts and nut butters
- Seeds
- Cheese (hard or soft)
- Vegetable-based soups
- Whole-grain crackers
- Popcorn
- Smoothies
- Hard-boiled eggs
- Cottage cheese

DINNER CHOICES

- Baked fish, poultry, or lean meat with vegetables
- Bean-based dishes
- Stir-fries
- Salads with fish, shellfish, or chicken
- Soup and salad
- Chili and salad
- Breakfast for dinner
- Open-faced sandwiches and soup or salad
- Re-created pizza, burritos, and casseroles

You've made some major changes in your weight and your health. Before you move on to the next stage of your life, I want you to pause for a few moments and give yourself some time to acknowledge your accomplishments. You have done some amazing things—you've lost weight, added healthy and delicious new foods to your diet, and taken charge of your health. I am so proud of you!

Earlier in the book we talked about how important it is to be mindful about what you eat. But it's also extremely valuable to be mindful of your achievements—the goals you've accomplished, the mountains you've climbed, the changes you've implemented, the successes you've experienced. Most of us have no problem dwelling on our missteps and weaknesses, but we often forget to celebrate our triumphs.

I want you to take a few minutes now to contemplate how much you have achieved as you've implemented The Doctor's Diet into your life. Write yourself a letter, or fill out the following worksheet. Doing so will help you really focus on the wonderful things you've accomplished!

MY AMAZING ACCOMPLISHMENTS WORKSHEET

I've lost _____ pounds.

I've lost _____ inches around my waist.

I have dropped _____ sizes and now wear a size _____.

I have lost my cravings for _____

_____.

I have discovered the following new foods and tastes that I love: _____

_____

_____

_____

_____

My blood pressure has improved. It was _____ , and now it's _____ .

My blood work/cholesterol/lipids are in a healthier range.
They are now:

_____

_____

_____

My blood sugar is lower. It was _____, and now it's _____.

Other positive changes I've noted (skin, hair, nails, libido, self-confidence, happiness, self-esteem, etc.) include:

_____

_____

_____

_____

_____

_____

_____

_____

My energy levels have changed. Now I feel: _____

_____

_____

_____

Next, take a moment to acknowledge the reasons that you want to continue living this new, healthy lifestyle and remain at this healthy weight. In other words, write something that inspires you to continue with your new lifestyle. Remember, my goal was to keep you out of the ER by lowering your weight and slashing your risk of developing chronic life-threatening diseases. What goals do you have for yourself?

_____

_____

_____

_____

_____

_____

_____

_____

Once you finish your Amazing Accomplishments Worksheet, post it where you can see it every day, or keep a copy in your smartphone. Reread it on a regular basis, and use it as a reminder of the path you've chosen to take.

During the STAT and RESTORE Plans, I gave you specific Meal Plan Equations to follow as you planned your meals. These equations were a great tool to help you focus on which foods to include in your healthy diet, as well as how much of those foods to eat for successful weight loss. But now that you've reached your weight-loss goals and become fully educated on the components of a healthy diet, you've become your own weight-loss expert. And when it comes to meal planning, I'm 100 percent confident that you're now ready to make your own choices about what to eat.

In the pages of this book, you've learned everything you need to know about nutrition, weight loss, and eating to reduce disease risk. As a result, you are well prepared to start making your own flexible choices about what to eat. You've graduated with honors and passed all of the tests: You understand what a healthy portion looks like. You know what kinds of foods foster robust health. You know which foods put your health in danger. You've had loads of practice creating balanced meals. Now, armed with information and experience, all you need is a healthy dose of common sense to guide you as you plan your MAINTAIN meals.

It's pretty simple. You're used to including a serving of lean protein at every meal, so continue to work that in. You're in the habit of eating two fruits daily, so stick with eating fruits and continue experimenting with different kinds. You're on top of the benefits of healthy fats, so continue to make smart choices about them. You're accustomed to filling your plate, bowl, and mug with Anytime Vegetables, Anytime Vegetable Soup, and Anytime Garden Salad, so keep up with that as well.

When it comes to carbohydrates, the best thing you can do for yourself is to follow my Carb-Flex approach. Here's how it works: Eat reasonable amounts of the healthiest carbs (carbohydrates from vegetables, fruits, legumes, whole grains), and avoid the not-so-good carbs (simple sugars from "white" foods, fruit juice, sweets, and candy). With the Carb-Flex approach, you use your activity levels to guide you as you make choices about carbohydrates. If you spent the morning hiking, for example, some extra complex carbohydrates are fine and sometimes necessary. But if you've been working late hours at the office and sitting around a lot with little or no exercise, go light on carbohydrates, choosing

Anytime Vegetables and keeping down to STAT-level amounts of whole grains. In other words, don't gobble down a whole-wheat dinner roll the size of your head at the end of a long day of sitting at your desk.

I do this in my own life. If I've been busy at work and haven't gotten a lot of activity in several days and I'm in the mood for a healthy Italian dish, rather than sitting down to a big bowl of whole-wheat pasta with chicken and veggies, I significantly reduce the amount of pasta I put in the bowl. I don't need those extra carbs because I'm not burning that much energy. Conversely, if I've been working out and hitting the trails on my bike and my activity level is through the roof, I might have a little extra whole-grain pasta because I know my body needs it to refuel.

I fully stand by my belief that your body needs complex carbohydrates and that they are good for you. But the reason why those "super low carb" diets work to help you shed pounds in a hurry is because carbohydrates are typical culprits of weight gain if you're not burning them off. So that's why I want your carbs to be your variable that changes based on your activity level. And the rule still applies—those simple, refined carbohydrates (white rice, white bread, regular pasta, sugary foods) really shouldn't have a place in your life, except for the occasional splurge.

MAINTAIN STRATEGY #3: EAT A WIDE VARIETY OF FOODS

There's a whole world of healthy, delicious, nutritious whole foods out there, and I want you to try as many of them as possible! They are packed with a world of nutrients—some of which we know about, some of which we don't. Experiment, and if you don't like something—well, then, try something else! Never stop being creative when it comes to nutritious foods.

For example, venture into the seafood aisle at the grocery store and try some kind of fish or shellfish that you haven't had before. Or, if you like wild game (or you want to see if you do), try duck, quail, goose, or pheasant. As for vegetables, check out all the bright, colorful, even exotic looking veggies at the store and give them a whirl. Same goes for fruit— you never know what kind of delicious delight you might find on the fruit stand.

To keep things interesting, use flavors that enliven your foods. Those flavors can come from herbs and spices, as well as various condiments, such as:

- Pickles
- Olives
- Mustards
- Cocktail sauce
- Pesto
- Relish

- Tabasco sauce
- Worcestershire sauce
- Chili paste
- Sesame tahini
- Salsa

MAINTAIN STRATEGY #4: RE-CREATE YOUR CRAVING FOODS

I love pizza. There's no way I'm going to give it up—and I wouldn't dream of asking you to give it up, either! The same goes for burritos, chicken parmesan, and a whole load of other foods generally considered not so healthy. The trick is not to walk away from these foods and never have them again. Nor is it to just give in and binge on them, gaining weight and accepting the fact that an elevated risk of disease is the price you have to pay to eat the foods you like.

You can keep on eating the foods you crave if you re-create them into healthy, good-for-you versions that will help you rather than work against you. This is absolutely what I do each and every day of my life. For example, instead of eating a day's worth of calories (and probably a week's worth of fat) with an extra-large pepperoni pizza from your local takeout place, make your own healthier version and eat it without guilt. The recipes in this book are a great place to start. You can also check out other cookbooks or online recipe sites for ideas.

Sure, it takes some imagination, time, and experimentation to re-create healthy versions of your favorite foods. You may end up with a few duds along the way—but hey, sometimes you have to kiss a few frogs before you find your prince or princess. And in the end, you'll end up with a list of re-created favorites that will be so tasty you won't even want to go back to the originals!

Here are a few ideas for re-created favorites:

- **Pizza:** Top a whole-wheat tortilla or whole-grain thin crust with tomato sauce, chopped veggies (onions, bell peppers, tomatoes, and mushrooms), shredded chicken, fresh or dried basil or oregano, and some grated Parmesan or feta cheese. Bake at 400 degrees until the cheese is melted.

- **Burritos:** Roll black beans, chopped tomatoes, cilantro, a squeeze of lime, grilled chicken breast, guacamole, chopped chili peppers, and your favorite salsa in a whole-grain tortilla—or spoon it all onto a bed of romaine lettuce and have a burrito bowl instead.

- **Chicken parmesan:** Spray chicken cutlets with cooking spray and coat with whole-grain bread crumbs. Place on a baking pan spritzed with cooking spray and bake for 20 minutes at 400 degrees. Top with tomato sauce, a sprinkle of Parmesan cheese, and serve with a small side of whole-grain pasta.

- **Seasoned French fries:** Cut two sweet potatoes into strips. Toss with a teaspoon of olive oil and a pinch of pepper, salt, chili powder, paprika, or whatever other low-sodium seasonings you like. Lay them out in a single layer on a sheet pan and bake at 450 degrees for about 20 minutes, or until crispy.

- **Rich chocolate dessert parfait:** Drizzle fresh fruit (berries, sliced peaches, mangoes, or bananas) with a small amount of honey. Mix 1 tablespoon dark chocolate chips (70 percent cocoa) into a cup of plain Greek yogurt. Layer the yogurt and the fruit in an elegant parfait glass.

Look for ways to make smart swaps as well. For example, if you like sour cream on a burrito, try mixing a little chili powder into plain Greek yogurt and plop that on instead. If you're in the mood for wings, grill some shrimp instead and brush it with buffalo sauce. And make a smart-carb swap by ALWAYS choosing "whole-grain" rather than "white" or "refined" when you're having cereal, tortillas, rice, pasta, or bread.

What will you re-create? Set goals for your top five former favorite cravings:

I used to crave: _____

_____

_____

How I can re-create it: _____

_____

_____

I used to crave: _____

_____

_____

How I can re-create it: _____

_____

_____

I used to crave: _____

_____

_____

How I can re-create it: _____

_____

_____

I used to crave: _____

_____

_____

How I can re-create it: _____

_____

_____

I used to crave: _____

_____

_____

How I can re-create it: _____

_____

_____

_____

MAINTAIN STRATEGY #5: WORK OFF YOUR SPLURGES

You can make some amazing re-creations of your favorite craving foods. The healthy pizza I make at home is way more delicious to me now than the greasy stuff in most pizza places. But I know that some foods can't be re-created. I completely understand that not every "unhealthy" urge you get can be redirected to a healthier version of that food. Most of the time there's some kind of healthier option, but it's unrealistic to expect 100 percent success.

My hope is that by the time you are starting with the MAINTAIN Plan, your standard cravings will be gone. By now, that giant slice of cheesecake probably doesn't appeal to you nearly as much as it used to. But if a splurge seems absolutely necessary for whatever reason, make a deal with yourself that you'll increase your activity level (even jogging in place while watching TV counts!) on the days that you just can't turn down the birthday cake, or you succumb to a croissant craving in the morning. If you're going to give in, then you should plan to "work it off" with some extra activity. Accountability is the key—when you give in to a splurge you don't feel guilt, but you *do* understand you need to be extra smart about food choices during the next day or two. After all, you don't want to lose all the progress you've made!

MAINTAIN STRATEGY #6: WEIGH YOURSELF ONCE A WEEK

I certainly don't want you to become obsessive about the number on your bathroom scale. But weighing yourself before you jump into the shower, say, every Wednesday morning, is a pretty good idea. This helps you see exactly how your eating habits affect your weight. If you notice that the number has crept up by five pounds or more, go back and do the STAT Plan for a week or two. If you're just three pounds above your goal weight, returning to RESTORE for a week or two should get you back on track. But if you're just up a little bit, then make a pact to cut down on carbohydrates, and you'll see a difference in no time. You have committed to a new way of life, one that's going to prolong your life and keep you out of the ER—so this little weekly check-in is a great reminder, and it'll be second nature before you know it.

MAINTAIN STRATEGY #7: MONITOR YOUR HEALTH

In addition to checking your weight weekly, pay attention to how your clothes are fitting, how you feel during exercise (and how often you're exercising), your blood pressure, and other measurements of health that your doctor can monitor for you. If you'd like, keep a daily or weekly journal, and jot down feelings, numbers, choices, and goals, so you always know how you're doing. And be sure to see your doctor as recommended for checkups.

MAINTAIN STRATEGY #8: MOVE, MOVE, MOVE!

When you commit to an active lifestyle, you not only boost your chances of keeping your weight off, but you experience a range of other health benefits, from better blood sugar and lower heart disease risk to an increase in energy and feelings of well-being. Exercise is the closest thing we have to a miracle for preventing the problems that send millions of people to the ER every year.

What's the best exercise for weight loss? Many studies have looked at this question. Although you might think the most strenuous activities—marathon running, cross-country skiing, long-distance biking, for example—are necessary for significant weight loss, that's not what many studies show. That's because it takes a lot of time and commitment to engage in marathon length activities. Also, people who engage in overly vigorous exercise are at risk for injuries.

The very best exercise for weight loss can really be anything—as long as you enjoy it and it suits your body's strengths and weaknesses. (If you've got a bum knee, for example, it's probably better to cycle than to run.) What matters for long-term weight maintenance is that you get out in the streets, into the gym, or over to the playing fields or courts most days of the week and do your activity for 30 to 60 minutes at an intensity that makes your heart rate go up.

When planning your activity, ask yourself what would make your exercise time so enjoyable that you'll look forward to it. Exercise is a drag when you're doing something you don't love, but if you pick something that revs your engines, you'll have no trouble staying motivated. Here are just a few examples:

+ If you love being with other people, join a fitness class.

+ If you want to raise money for a cause you believe in, train for a charity walk that supports that cause.

+ If great music jazzes you, sign up for a dance class.

+ If you want to challenge yourself, commit to a race and train for it.

+ If you're the solitary type, go running in the morning.

+ If you're interested in learning a new sport or activity, sign up for lessons at your local Y or through your town's park and rec department.

+ If you're competitive, play a sport.

+ If you don't like sweating, go swimming.

+ If you like catching up with friends, walk with a different one every morning of the week.

+ If you need an escape at lunchtime, take a midday yoga class.

+ If you need more time with your spouse, take long bike rides together on the weekends.

+ If you love the great outdoors, go hiking.

+ If you have the time, safe paths, and a place to shower in the morning, ride your bike to work.

+ If you love hiking and biking, plan an active vacation that you spend moving through the mountains rather than lying by the pool.

✚ Or combine a bunch of activities you like—it doesn't really matter what you do, as long as you're moving your body on an almost-every-day basis.

Whether you choose walking, jogging, biking, swimming, skiing, group exercise classes, exercise machines in the gym, yoga, lifting weights, playing tennis, joining a team sport, or anything else at all, you will get huge benefits if you make physical activity part of your daily life. Design your daily life in such a way that movement is incorporated. Include cardio, resistance, and flexibility activities in your program.

Finally, make sure to work activity into every part of your day. Take the stairs instead of the elevator, park your car farther from your destination, ride your bike to the store instead of driving, stand more than you sit—you know what to do.

✚ MAKE HEALTH AND HEALTHY EATING YOUR HOBBY FOR THE REST OF YOUR LIFE! AND INSPIRE OTHERS TO DO THE SAME!

CONCLUSION

In the end, the ultimate MAINTAIN strategy of all is to make health your hobby. Good health can be the foundation for a wonderful life and I hope this book has provided some ideas on how to build that foundation. I started this book with some scary statistics about how the food we eat can cause illness and ultimately a visit to the emergency room or an untimely death. But hopefully you now understand the opposite is also true: food truly can be our medicine. The kind of medicine that requires no prescription and that you can enjoy for the rest of your long, happy and healthy life. Good luck on your journey and may you inspire many others along the way. I'll be rooting for you!

THE DOCTOR'S DIET RECIPE GUIDE

BREAKFAST RECIPES

Breakfast recipes each contain 1 **Breakfast Protein**.

Some contain **1 STAT Fruit, 1 Other Fruit**, or **Anytime Vegetables**.

Flex-Time Foods are listed as optional ingredients.

Unless otherwise indicated, recipes fit all plans
(**STAT**, **RESTORE**, and **MAINTAIN**).

BERRY SMOOTHIE

1 cup milk or yogurt

1 cup frozen berries

Place all ingredients in a blender. Blend together until smooth. Makes
1 serving.

BANANA SMOOTHIE
(RESTORE and MAINTAIN only)

1 cup milk or yogurt

1 small banana

Several ice cubes

Place all ingredients in a blender. Blend together until smooth. Makes 1 serving.

VEGGIE SMOOTHIE

1 cup milk or yogurt

1 cup frozen berries (optional for RESTORE and MAINTAIN: substitute 1 small banana, 1 cup chopped fresh peaches, or other soft fruit)

1 handful baby spinach leaves

Optional: 1 teaspoon honey

Place all ingredients in a blender. Blend together until smooth. Makes 1 serving.

NUTTY-BERRY SMOOTHIE

½ cup milk or yogurt

1 cup frozen berries (optional for RESTORE and MAINTAIN: substitute 1 small banana, 1 cup chopped fresh peaches, or other soft fruit)

½ tablespoon nut butter

Place all ingredients in a blender. Blend together until smooth. Makes 1 serving.

HIGH-PROTEIN BREAKFAST SMOOTHIE

1 cup milk or yogurt

1 cup frozen berries (optional for RESTORE and MAINTAIN: substitute 1 small banana, 1 cup chopped fresh peaches, or other soft fruit)

1 scoop protein powder (such as whey, brown-rice protein, or hemp protein)

Optional: ½ cup oatmeal

Place all ingredients in a blender. Blend together until smooth. Makes 1 serving.

MEDITERRANEAN SKILLET SCRAMBLE

Olive oil cooking spray

¼ cup onion, diced

¼ cup tomato, diced

¼ cup zucchini, diced

1 egg or 3 egg whites, beaten

Fresh or dried basil and/or oregano

2–4 black or green olives, sliced or diced

Coat a small skillet with olive oil cooking spray. Sauté onions, tomato, and zucchini until veggies are soft. Pour egg over the vegetables. Sprinkle with herbs and stir slowly while cooking. Flip and cook to desired doneness. Top with olives. Makes 1 serving.

SPINACH OMELET

Olive oil cooking spray

¼ cup onion, diced

Handful of baby spinach leaves

1 egg or 3 egg whites

Dash of nutmeg

Coat a small skillet with the olive oil cooking spray. Sauté onions and spinach until veggies are soft. Pour egg over the vegetables. Sprinkle in nutmeg and stir slowly while cooking. Flip and cook to desired doneness. Makes 1 serving.

MUSHROOM OMELET

Olive oil cooking spray

¼ cup onion, diced

½ cup white mushrooms, sliced

1 egg or 3 egg whites

Black pepper

Coat a small skillet with the olive oil cooking spray. Sauté onions and mushrooms until veggies are soft. Pour egg over the vegetables. Stir slowly while cooking. Flip and cook to desired doneness. Pepper to taste. Makes 1 serving.

CHEESY BROCCOLI OMELET

Olive oil cooking spray

¼ cup onion, diced

½ cup broccoli florets, chopped into small pieces

3 egg whites

1 ounce cheddar cheese, shredded

Coat a small skillet with the olive oil cooking spray. Sauté onions and broccoli until veggies are soft. Pour egg over vegetables. Stir slowly while cooking. Flip and cook until almost done. Top with shredded cheese; fold in half so cheese is enclosed and continue to cook until cheese is melted and eggs are done. Makes 1 serving.

BANANA-EGG PANCAKES
(RESTORE and MAINTAIN only)

1 egg, whisked well

1 small banana, very ripe, mashed well

Sprinkle of cinnamon

Olive oil cooking spray

Optional: 1 cup mixed berries

Combine egg, banana, and cinnamon and mix well. Coat a skillet with olive oil cooking spray and set over medium heat. When skillet is medium-hot, pour batter into pan. When bottom side of pancake is cooked, flip and continue cooking until done. Top with berries and serve.

BREAKFAST BANANA SPLIT
(RESTORE and MAINTAIN only)

½ small banana, peeled and cut lengthwise

1 cup of low-fat Greek yogurt (plain)

½ cup strawberries or raspberries, sliced

Optional: Handful of chopped walnuts

Place the banana on a plate. Top with yogurt, berries, and nuts (if using). Makes 1 serving.

MAIN-DISH RECIPES

Main-dish recipes contain 1 Main-Dish Protein per serving.

Many contain Anytime Vegetables.

Flex-Time Foods are listed as optional ingredients.

Unless otherwise indicated, recipes fit all plans
(STAT, RESTORE, and MAINTAIN).

MAIN-DISH SALADS

For Versatile Vinaigrette recipe, see page 244.

GARBANZO BEAN SALAD

½ cup garbanzo beans, drained

½ cup cucumber, chopped

2 tablespoons red onion, chopped

1 teaspoon garlic, minced

Fresh chopped parsley to taste

Dash of pepper

Balsamic vinegar

1 large tomato, sliced

Optional: 1½ tablespoons Versatile Vinaigrette

Toss all ingredients together except tomato slices. Spritz with olive oil cooking spray and drizzle with a little balsamic vinegar, or dress with Versatile Vinaigrette. Serve over tomato slices. Makes 1 serving.

VERSATILE VINAIGRETTE

⅓ cup any kind of vinegar (balsamic, white, cider, red wine, etc.)

1 teaspoon honey (optional)

1 teaspoon lemon, lime, orange, grapefruit, mango, pineapple, or other fruit juice (or for a richer taste, add 1 tablespoon tomato juice, vegetable juice, or tomato sauce)

1 teaspoon garlic (or more to taste), minced

1 teaspoon onions or shallots (optional), minced

Chopped fresh or dried herbs to taste (basil, thyme, rosemary, parsley, sage, lemongrass, cilantro, etc.)

Salt and pepper to taste

⅔ cup extra-virgin olive oil

Whisk together vinegar, honey, fruit or vegetable juice, garlic, onions or shallots if using, herbs, and salt and pepper. To create an emulsified dressing (the oil and vinegar stay combined), slowly pour olive oil into the vinegar mixture in a very thin stream while whisking vigorously. You can also use a food processor, or just combine all the ingredients in a jar and shake well before using. Makes about 10–12 servings of 1½ tablespoons each.

BABY SPINACH SALAD

1–2 cups baby spinach leaves

½ cup grape tomatoes, sliced

2 tablespoons onion, chopped

1 hard-boiled egg or 3 hard-boiled egg whites, chopped

1 ounce crumbled low-fat feta cheese

Olive oil cooking spray

Balsamic vinegar

Optional: 1½ tablespoons Versatile Vinaigrette

Arrange spinach leaves on a plate. Top with tomatoes, onion, eggs or egg whites, and cheese. Spritz with olive oil cooking spray and drizzle with a little balsamic vinegar, or dress with Versatile Vinaigrette. Makes 1 serving.

TUNA ROMAINE SALAD

1–2 cups romaine lettuce

3–4 ounces canned tuna packed in water, drained

½ cup cooked green beans, chilled

½ cup grape tomatoes, sliced

Olive oil cooking spray

Balsamic vinegar

Optional: 1½ tablespoons Versatile Vinaigrette

Arrange lettuce leaves on a plate. Top with tuna, green beans, and tomatoes. Spritz with olive oil cooking spray and drizzle with a little balsamic vinegar, or dress with Versatile Vinaigrette. Makes 1 serving.

TUNA BEAN SALAD

1–2 cups romaine lettuce

2 ounces canned tuna packed in water, drained

½ cup cooked white beans

½ cup cooked green beans, chilled

½ cup grape tomatoes, sliced

Fresh chopped herbs to taste

Olive oil cooking spray

Balsamic vinegar

Optional: 1½ tablespoons Versatile Vinaigrette

Arrange lettuce leaves on a plate. Top with tuna, white beans, green beans, tomatoes, and herbs. Spritz with olive oil cooking spray and drizzle with a little balsamic vinegar, or dress with Versatile Vinaigrette. Makes 1 serving.

TUNA SANDWICH SALAD

3–4 ounces canned tuna packed in water, drained

1 tablespoon celery, chopped

1 tablespoon dill relish, or 1 tablespoon chopped dill pickle

1 tablespoon plain Greek yogurt

½ teaspoon Dijon mustard

1 slice of tomato

Optional: 1 slice of whole-grain bread, toasted

Optional: 1–2 cups salad greens

Mix together tuna, celery, relish or pickle, yogurt, and mustard. Arrange slice of tomato on the toast (for an open-faced sandwich) or the salad greens (for a salad). Top with tuna mixture. Makes 1 serving.

TEX-MEX SALAD

1–2 cups salad greens, any type

¼ cup black beans, drained

½ teaspoon cumin

½ cup fresh salsa

1 ounce cheddar cheese, shredded

Optional: ½ small avocado, cubed

Arrange salad greens on a plate. Spread with black beans. Mix cumin into salsa; pour over beans. Top with shredded cheddar cheese and avocado (if using). Makes 1 serving.

GREEK LENTIL SALAD

1–2 cups baby spinach leaves

½ cup cooked and chilled lentils

½ cucumber, diced

5 grape tomatoes, sliced

1 ounce feta cheese

Olive oil cooking spray

Balsamic vinegar

Optional: 1½ tablespoons Versatile Vinaigrette

Arrange spinach leaves on a plate. Mix together lentils and cucumber and place on spinach. Top with the grape tomatoes and cheese. Spritz with olive oil cooking spray and drizzle with a little balsamic vinegar, or dress with Versatile Vinaigrette. Makes 1 serving.

TUSCAN BEAN SALAD

¼ cup white beans, rinsed and drained

¼ cup kidney beans, rinsed and drained (or use ½ cup all white beans)

¼ cup red onion, chopped

½ cup grape tomatoes, sliced

Chopped fresh parsley

1 tablespoon balsamic vinegar

1–2 cups salad greens, any type

4 black or green olives, sliced

Optional: 1 tablespoon olive oil

Mix beans, onion, tomatoes, and parsley. Toss with vinegar and olive oil (if using). Arrange bean mixture over salad greens and top with olives. Makes 1 serving.

VEGETABLE AND CHEESE SALAD WITH PECANS

1 medium tomato, diced

½ cucumber, diced

½ green pepper, diced

1 ounce cheddar cheese, cubed or shredded

Handful (½ ounce) of chopped pecans

Fresh parsley, thyme, or other herbs, chopped

1–2 cups salad greens, any type

Olive oil cooking spray

Balsamic vinegar

Optional: 1½ tablespoons Versatile Vinaigrette

Toss together all ingredients. Spritz with olive oil cooking spray and drizzle with a little balsamic vinegar, or dress with Versatile Vinaigrette. Makes 1 serving.

CAPRESE SALAD

1–2 cups salad greens, any type, shredded

1 tomato, sliced

¼ cup thinly cut red onion slices

2 ounces fresh mozzarella balls

Fresh basil leaves, shredded

Olive oil cooking spray

Balsamic vinegar

Optional: 1½ tablespoons Versatile Vinaigrette

On salad greens, place tomato slices, onion slices, mozzarella balls, and basil leaves. Spritz with olive oil cooking spray and drizzle with a little balsamic vinegar, or dress with Versatile Vinaigrette. Makes 1 serving.

CAESAR SALAD WITH CHICKEN, SALMON, OR SHRIMP

1–2 cups romaine lettuce, shredded

3-4 ounces grilled or baked chicken, salmon, or shrimp

2 tablespoons onion, chopped

½ cup roasted red pepper (packed in water), chopped

½ ounce fresh Parmesan cheese, shredded or thinly sliced

Olive oil cooking spray

Balsamic vinegar

Optional: 1½ tablespoons Versatile Vinaigrette

Optional: Garlic Croutons (see recipe)

Arrange lettuce leaves on a plate. Top with chicken, salmon, or shrimp; onion; roasted red peppers; and cheese. Spritz with olive oil cooking spray and drizzle with a little balsamic vinegar, or dress with Versatile Vinaigrette. Top with Garlic Croutons (if using). Makes 1 serving.

GARLIC CROUTONS

1 slice whole-grain bread

Olive oil cooking spray

1 tablespoon chopped garlic, or ¼ teaspoon garlic powder

Spritz bread on both sides with olive oil cooking spray. Toast one side under broiler until brown. Flip over, top with garlic or garlic powder, and toast under broiler until brown. Cut up into squares. Makes 1 serving.

CHEF SALAD

1–2 cups salad greens, any type

2 ounces baked chicken breast, cut in strips

½ tomato, chopped

1 ounce cheddar cheese, shredded or cubed

2 hard-boiled egg whites, chopped

Black pepper

Olive oil cooking spray

Balsamic vinegar

Optional: 1½ tablespoons Versatile Vinaigrette

Arrange salad greens on a plate. Top with chicken, tomato, cheese, and egg whites. Sprinkle with black pepper. Spritz with olive oil cooking spray and drizzle with a little balsamic vinegar, or dress with Versatile Vinaigrette. Makes 1 serving.

QUICK-FIX BEAN BURRITO BOWL SALAD

1–2 cups salad greens, shredded

¼ cup canned black beans, drained

2 tablespoons canned chopped green chilies, or more to taste

¼ cup salsa, fresh or bottled

1 ounce cheddar cheese, shredded

Optional: ¼ cup guacamole

Optional: 1 whole-grain tortilla

Arrange salad greens in a bowl. Top with beans, green chilies, salsa, cheese, and guacamole (if using) or roll into tortilla. Makes 1 serving.

CHICKEN AND RICE SALAD

3–4 ounces cooked chicken breast, cubed

Optional: ½ cup brown rice, cooked

1 tablespoon olive oil

¼ to ½ teaspoon turmeric or curry powder

1–2 cups salad greens, any type, shredded

1 tomato, sliced

Olive oil cooking spray

Cider vinegar

Optional: 1½ tablespoons Versatile Vinaigrette

In a small bowl, mix together chicken, rice (if using), olive oil, and turmeric or curry powder. Arrange salad greens on a plate. Top with tomato slices. Place chicken mixture over the tomato. Spritz with olive oil cooking spray and splash with a little cider vinegar, or dress with Versatile Vinaigrette. Makes 1 serving.

MEATLESS CHEF SALAD

1–2 cups salad greens, any type

½ tomato, chopped

1 ounce cheddar cheese, grated

¼ cup cooked lentils

Olive oil cooking spray

Cider vinegar

Optional: ½ small avocado, sliced

Optional: 1½ tablespoons Versatile Vinaigrette

Arrange salad greens on a plate. Top with tomato, cheese, lentils, and avocado (if using). Spritz with olive oil cooking spray and splash with a little cider vinegar, or dress with Versatile Vinaigrette. Makes 1 serving.

TABBOULEH AND FETA

⅔ cup bulgur wheat

1 tablespoon lemon juice

⅔ cup boiling water

2 medium tomatoes, chopped

2 green onions, sliced

½ cup fresh parsley, chopped

2 tablespoons fresh mint, chopped

Olive oil cooking spray

4 ounces feta cheese

Lettuce leaves

Optional: 1½ tablespoons Versatile Vinaigrette

Combine the bulgur, lemon juice, and boiling water. Let this mixture stand about 30 minutes, allowing bulgur to absorb the liquid. Stir in tomatoes, green onions, parsley, and mint. Spray with olive oil cooking spray (or dress with Versatile Vinaigrette) and gently toss in the feta cheese. Chill for at least 1 hour. Arrange the mixture over lettuce leaves. Makes 4 servings.

MAIN-DISH SOUPS AND CHILIES

LENTIL SOUP

Olive oil cooking spray

1 medium onion, chopped

2 stalks celery, diced

2 carrots, diced

1 small garlic clove, minced

32-ounce box fat-free, reduced-sodium chicken, beef, or vegetable broth

15-ounce can crushed or diced tomatoes, or 15-ounce can tomato sauce

1 cup dry lentils

1 cup baby spinach, sliced thin

1 teaspoon vinegar

½ teaspoon cumin

1 teaspoon dried oregano

1 bay leaf

Dash of freshly ground black pepper

Spray a saucepan with olive oil cooking spray and heat on medium. Add onion, celery, and carrots, sautéing for a few minutes, until they start to soften. Add garlic and sauté for another minute. Add in all remaining ingredients. Bring to a boil. Reduce heat to low, cover, and simmer gently for 25 to 35 minutes, or until lentils are tender. Remove bay leaf before serving. If soup is thicker than you like, thin with water. Makes 6 servings.

MINESTRONE SOUP

1 32-ounce box fat-free, reduced-sodium chicken or vegetable broth

1 15-ounce can crushed tomatoes

2 zucchinis, quartered and sliced

1 tablespoon garlic, minced

1 large onion, chopped

2 stalks celery, chopped

2 carrots, sliced

2 cups canned kidney beans, drained

1 cup frozen green beans

2 teaspoons dried oregano

2 teaspoons dried basil

Parmesan cheese

In a large saucepan or soup pot, combine broth, tomatoes, zucchini, garlic, onion, celery, and carrots. Bring to a boil; cover and reduce heat. Simmer until vegetables are tender, about 20 minutes. Add kidney beans, green beans, oregano, and basil. Simmer for 5–8 minutes, until green beans are tender. Top each serving with a sprinkle of Parmesan cheese prior to serving. Makes 4 servings.

BEEFY BEAN AND VEGETABLE SOUP

Olive oil cooking spray

1 medium onion, chopped

2 stalks celery, diced

2 carrots, diced

1 32-ounce box fat-free, reduced-sodium beef broth

1 15-ounce can tomato sauce

1 tablespoon Tabasco sauce

8 ounces cooked roast beef, cut into small pieces

1 bay leaf

1 cup canned kidney beans, drained

Dash of freshly ground black pepper

Spray a saucepan with olive oil cooking spray and heat on medium. Add onion, celery, and carrots, sautéing for a few minutes, until they start to soften. Add in all remaining ingredients except beans. Bring to a boil. Reduce heat to low, cover, and simmer gently for 20 minutes. Add beans and simmer 10 minutes longer. Remove bay leaf before serving. Makes 6 servings.

TURKEY BLACK BEAN CHILI

Olive oil cooking spray

½ pound lean ground turkey

1 medium onion, chopped

1 red bell pepper, chopped

1 cup canned black beans, drained

½ cup chunky salsa

2 cups crushed tomato

1 tablespoon chili powder

1 teaspoon cumin

½ teaspoon garlic powder

¼ teaspoon pepper

Spray a large skillet with olive oil cooking spray. Brown the turkey along with the onions and peppers over medium heat. Add the rest of the ingredients and heat until bubbling. Reduce heat and simmer, covered, for 30 minutes. Makes 4 servings.

OLD WEST CHILI

Olive oil cooking spray

1 pound ground buffalo meat or lean beef

1 large onion, chopped

1 green bell pepper, chopped

1 tablespoon garlic, minced

1 15-ounce can crushed tomatoes

2 cups fat-free beef broth

1 tablespoon chili powder

1 teaspoon cumin

½ teaspoon red pepper flakes

Spray a large skillet with olive oil cooking spray. Brown buffalo meat or beef and pour off any residual fat. Add the onion, green bell pepper, and garlic. Cook until soft. Add the rest of the ingredients and heat until bubbling. Reduce heat and simmer, covered, for 30 minutes. Makes 4 servings.

ANYTIME VEGETABLE SOUP

One cup of this soup contains a full serving (or more!) of Anytime Vegetables. Cook a big batch and freeze it in microwaveable one-cup containers; you can heat it up in minutes for lunch, dinner, or a snack.

Olive oil cooking spray

½ cup onions, chopped

1 small garlic clove, minced

1 cup celery, chopped

1 cup carrots, chopped

1 cup spinach or cabbage, sliced thin

½ cup of any kind of Anytime Vegetables, such as green beans, broccoli, cauliflower, mushrooms, squash, or wax beans

1 32-ounce box fat-free, reduced-sodium chicken, beef, or vegetable broth

1 15-ounce can crushed or diced tomatoes, or 15-ounce can tomato sauce

Dash of freshly ground black pepper

Fresh or dried parsley, basil, oregano, or other herbs, to taste

Spray a saucepan with cooking spray and heat on medium. Add onion, garlic, celery, carrots, spinach, cabbage, and your choice of Anytime Vegetables, sautéing for a few minutes, until they start to soften. Add broth, tomatoes or tomato sauce, herbs, and pepper. Bring to a boil. Reduce heat to low, cover, and simmer for 20–30 minutes, or until the vegetables are cooked to the doneness you like. Makes 6 or more servings, depending on how many vegetables you add.

ANYTIME GARDEN SALAD

Have this salad anytime you want—it's full of Anytime Vegetables. If you'd like to use your daily Flex-Time Healthy Fat choice with your salad, choose 1½ tablespoons of my Versatile Vinaigrette. If not, give your salad a spritz of olive oil cooking spray and a splash of vinegar. Or top it with a scoop of fresh salsa.

Place 1–2 cups spinach, romaine, or any other salad greens in a bowl. Top with your choice of raw vegetables, including chopped or sliced tomatoes, celery, bell peppers, broccoli or cauliflower florets, red cabbage, cucumbers, jicama, mushrooms, onions, pea pods, or radishes. You can also throw in your choice of cooked leftover vegetables, such as sautéed peppers, green beans, roasted eggplant, sautéed mushrooms, roasted squash, and wax beans.

Optional add-ins: Healthy Fats (½ small avocado or ¼ cup guacamole) or Snack Proteins (handful of nuts, handful of seeds, 1 ounce shredded sharp cheese, ½ cup cottage cheese, or 1 ounce feta cheese).

ANYTIME SALSA

2 15-ounce cans petite diced tomatoes, drained, juice reserved

1 medium onion, yellow or red, chopped

2–4 garlic cloves, minced

Juice of 1 small lime

1 jalapeño pepper, seeds removed, minced

¼ cup fresh cilantro, chopped

Combine all ingredients in a bowl. Mash with a potato masher or fork if desired. (Alternately, roughly chop ingredients in a food processor.) Add in reserved juice until the salsa reaches desired consistency.

DILL SALMON

1 pound salmon (4 fillets)

Olive oil cooking spray

1 tablespoon chopped fresh or dried dill

½ teaspoon garlic powder

¼ teaspoon black pepper

2 teaspoons lemon juice, fresh or bottled

Preheat oven to 350 degrees. Place salmon fillets in a glass baking dish that has been lightly coated with olive oil cooking spray. In a small bowl, mix together the herbs and spices. Season the salmon with the herb and spice mixture. Spray the fillets lightly with olive oil cooking spray. Sprinkle lemon juice over fillets. Bake 25 minutes, or until salmon flakes easily with a fork. Makes 4 servings.

LEMON-ROSEMARY SALMON

1 pound salmon (4 fillets)

Olive oil cooking spray

1 tablespoon fresh rosemary leaves, chopped fine

Juice of two lemons

Preheat oven to 350 degrees. Place salmon fillets in a glass baking dish that has been lightly coated with olive oil cooking spray. Spray the fillets lightly with olive oil cooking spray, then sprinkle with lemon juice and rosemary. Bake 25 minutes, or until salmon flakes easily with a fork. Makes 4 servings.

CURRIED TILAPIA

1 teaspoon paprika

1 teaspoon curry powder

1 pound tilapia (4 fillets)

Olive oil cooking spray

2 teaspoons lemon juice, fresh or bottled

Preheat oven to 400 degrees. Mix together the paprika and curry powder. Rub the spice mixture on the fish fillets. Spray fillets lightly with olive oil cooking spray; place them in a glass baking dish that has been lightly coated with olive oil cooking spray. Bake at 400 degrees for 15–20 minutes, or until fish flakes easily with a fork. Sprinkle with the lemon juice and serve. Makes 4 servings.

BAKED COD WITH TOMATOES

1 pound cod or other white fish (4 fillets)

Olive oil cooking spray

3 plum tomatoes, thinly sliced

2 garlic cloves, minced

1 teaspoon dried oregano

Preheat oven to 400 degrees. Spray fillets lightly with olive oil cooking spray; place them in a glass baking dish that has been lightly coated with olive oil cooking spray. Top with tomato slices; sprinkle with garlic and oregano. Bake at 400 degrees for 15–20 minutes, or until fish flakes easily with a fork. Makes 4 servings.

SCALLOP KABOBS

1 pound scallops, raw

1 medium yellow bell pepper, cut into bite-sized chunks

1 medium green bell pepper, cut into bite-sized chunks

8 cherry tomatoes

8 white pearl onions

Olive oil cooking spray

Balsamic vinegar

Thread scallops, pepper chunks, cherry tomatoes, and onions on kabob skewers. Spray with olive oil cooking spray, then brush with balsamic vinegar. Grill over a medium flame for about 20 minutes, brushing with extra vinegar. Makes 4 servings.

GARLIC SHRIMP

Olive oil cooking spray

1 pound large uncooked shrimp, shelled and deveined

2 garlic cloves, minced

1 tablespoon honey

¼ cup dry white wine

In a skillet coated with olive oil cooking spray, sauté shrimp and garlic until shrimp is cooked. Add honey and wine. Simmer for 5–6 minutes, or until marmalade mixture has thickened. Makes 4 servings.

SPAGHETTI SQUASH WITH MEAT SAUCE

1 spaghetti squash

Olive oil cooking spray

1 pound lean ground turkey or buffalo meat

1 28-ounce can peeled, crushed tomatoes

2 teaspoons dried Italian herbs, or 1 teaspoon each dried basil and oregano

2 garlic cloves, minced

Parmesan cheese

Preheat oven to 400 degrees. Cut squash in half lengthwise. Place in a baking dish, cut-side up, with 1 inch of water. Bake for 45 minutes, or until squash is tender. Meanwhile, in a skillet spritzed with olive oil cooking spray, brown the meat until fully cooked. Stir in tomatoes, herbs, and garlic. Simmer over low heat until the squash is ready. When the squash is finished cooking, use a fork to pull out strands of the squash. Discard seeds. Pour the meat sauce over the squash, sprinkle with Parmesan cheese, and serve. Makes 4 servings.

MAIN-DISH ROAST BEEF SALAD

Olive oil cooking spray

1 pound sirloin steak, visible fat trimmed

2 tablespoons fish sauce

1 teaspoon honey

1 garlic clove, minced

¼ teaspoon red pepper flakes

Juice of 1 lime

1 head of Boston lettuce, torn into bite-sized pieces

1 medium red bell pepper, seeded and cut into strips

2 carrots, cut into matchstick pieces

3 green onions, chopped

½ cup of cilantro, shredded

In a skillet that has been coated with olive oil cooking spray, sauté the beef to desired doneness. Remove from pan; slice the beef into thin slices at an angle. To make the dressing, whisk together fish sauce, honey, garlic, red pepper flakes, and lime juice in a small bowl. Arrange lettuce on four plates. Top with equal portions of red bell pepper, carrots, green onions, and cilantro. Place equal portions of the sliced beef atop the vegetables. Drizzle the dressing over each serving. Makes 4 servings.

MEATZA PIZZA

1 pound extra-lean ground beef

1 egg

1 teaspoon dried Italian spices

1 teaspoon garlic powder

½ teaspoon black pepper

¼ cup Parmesan cheese

Olive oil cooking spray

½ cup tomato sauce

½ cup chopped fresh tomatoes

½ cup onions, chopped

½ cup zucchini, chopped

½ cup shredded part-skim mozzarella cheese

Preheat oven to 450 degrees. Mix the ground beef, egg, garlic, pepper, and Italian spices in a mixing bowl until thoroughly incorporated. Add Parmesan cheese; mix well. Press beef mixture evenly onto a baking pan that has been coated with olive cooking spray. Bake about 20 minutes, until meat is browned. Remove from the oven and drain off any residual fat. Spread the tomato sauce around the "crust." Arrange tomatoes, onions, and zucchini on top. Sprinkle mozzarella cheese over vegetables. Return to the oven and bake for an additional 20 minutes, or until vegetables are soft. Makes 4 servings.

PORK KABOBS

1 pound boneless loin pork chops, cut into 1-inch cubes

1 medium red bell pepper, cut into bite-sized chunks

1 medium green bell pepper, cut into bite-sized chunks

1 red onion, cut into 1-inch pieces

1 tablespoon sesame oil

1 tablespoon soy sauce

Black pepper

Optional: 1 cup fresh pineapple, cut into 1-inch chunks

Thread pork, pepper chunks, red onion, and pineapple (if using) on kabob skewers. Mix sesame oil and soy sauce; brush onto skewers. Sprinkle with black pepper. Grill over a medium flame until pork is cooked through, approximately 8–12 minutes. Makes 4 servings.

BEEF SKILLET STEW

Olive oil cooking spray

1 pound boneless sirloin steak or round steak, fat removed, cut into bite-size pieces

1 onion, chopped

1 cup mushrooms

1 cup fat-free, reduced-sodium beef broth

1 cup tomato sauce, tomato juice, or vegetable juice

1 tablespoon Worcestershire sauce

1 bay leaf

1 teaspoon dried thyme leaves

1 teaspoon dried rosemary leaves, crumbled

2 tablespoons dried parsley

3 carrots, chopped

4 celery stalks, chopped

1 cup green beans, chopped

1 tablespoon cornstarch mixed well with 2 tablespoons beef broth
or water

In a large skillet sprayed with olive oil cooking spray, sauté beef, onions, and mushrooms until beef is brown. Add beef broth, tomato sauce or juice, Worcestershire sauce, and herbs; heat until bubbly. Reduce heat to low, cover, and simmer for 30 minutes, stirring occasionally. Add carrots, celery, and green beans and simmer for 30 more minutes. Add cornstarch-broth mixture, stir well, and heat for 3–5 more minutes, until thickened. Remove bay leaf before serving. Serves 4.

BAKED GINGER-MARINATED PORK OR CHICKEN

1 pound boneless pork chops, fat removed (or 1 pound boneless, skinless chicken breasts)

2 tablespoons low-sodium soy sauce

2 tablespoons tomato paste

2 tablespoons fresh ginger, grated

2 garlic cloves, minced

1 tablespoon honey

1 tablespoon cider vinegar

Combine soy sauce, tomato paste, ginger, garlic, honey, and vinegar in a bowl with pork chops. Marinate for 30–60 minutes in a ceramic or glass baking dish. Heat oven to 375 degrees. Place dish in oven and bake 30–40 minutes, or until pork chops are cooked through. Serve with sauce on the side.

SALSA CHICKEN

1 cup salsa, fresh or bottled

1 teaspoon cumin

1 teaspoon chili powder

1 tablespoon fresh lime juice

1 pound skinless, boneless chicken breasts

Olive oil cooking spray

Fresh cilantro, chopped

Preheat oven to 375 degrees. In a bowl, combine salsa, cumin, chili powder, and fresh lime juice. Place chicken in a baking dish that has been sprayed with olive oil cooking spray. Pour salsa mixture over chicken, flipping chicken until well coated with salsa. Bake 20–30 minutes, or until chicken is cooked through. During cooking, baste chicken occasionally with salsa. Top with fresh cilantro. Makes 4 servings.

CHICKEN PARMESAN

1 cup of Parmesan cheese, divided

1 teaspoon oregano

½ teaspoon garlic powder

1 pound skinless, boneless chicken breasts

4 egg whites, beaten

Olive oil cooking spray

Terrific Tomato Sauce (see recipe)

Preheat oven to 350 degrees. Mix ¾ cup Parmesan cheese, oregano, and garlic powder; spread out on a plate. Dip each chicken breast, one by one, in the beaten egg white mixture, then roll in the cheese mixture. Place the coated chicken breasts in a baking dish that has been sprayed with olive oil cooking spray. Spritz chicken breasts lightly with cooking spray. Bake for 45 minutes. Serve each chicken breast with Terrific Tomato Sauce; sprinkle with the remaining ¼ cup Parmesan cheese.

TERRIFIC TOMATO SAUCE

1 tablespoon olive oil

1 onion, chopped

2 garlic cloves, minced

1 28-ounce can peeled, ground tomatoes

1 teaspoon dried oregano

1 teaspoon dried basil

1 tablespoon balsamic vinegar

2 tablespoons tomato paste

In a medium saucepan, heat olive oil. Sauté onion and garlic for 2–3 minutes, until they start to soften. Stir in tomatoes, oregano, basil, vinegar, and tomato paste. Heat to bubbling; cover, reduce heat, and simmer 15 minutes. Makes 6–8 half-cup servings.

EGGPLANT PARMESAN

1 large eggplant, peeled

½ cup whole-wheat panko breadcrumbs

1 cup Parmesan cheese, divided

1 teaspoon garlic powder

2 teaspoons dried Italian herbs

2 egg whites, beaten

Olive oil cooking spray

1 cup Terrific Tomato Sauce (see recipe)

Preheat oven to 400 degrees. Cut eggplant lengthwise into 4 thick strips. Combine breadcrumbs, ¾ cup of the Parmesan cheese, garlic, and herbs in a shallow bowl. Whisk egg whites in another shallow bowl. Dip eggplant slices into egg whites, then roll each strip in bread-crumb-cheese mixture. Place eggplant on cooking sheet that has been sprayed with olive oil spray. Spray olive oil spray over eggplant slices. Bake 30 minutes, or until nice and brown on top and cooked through. Spread Terrific Tomato Sauce over the eggplant; return to oven and bake for another 20 minutes. Sprinkle with remaining ¼ cup Parmesan cheese before serving. Makes 2 main-dish servings or 4 side-dish servings.

CHICKEN, BEEF, PORK, OR SHRIMP STIR-FRY

Olive oil cooking spray

1 pound chicken, beef, or pork, cut into bite-size pieces, or 1 pound shrimp

1 red pepper, cut in 1-inch strips

1 yellow pepper, cut in 1-inch strips

1 green pepper, cut in 1-inch strips

1 cup broccoli florets, chopped

3 celery stalks, chopped

1 cup bean sprouts

½ cup fat-free, reduced-sodium chicken, beef, or vegetable broth

2 tablespoons low-sodium soy sauce

1 tablespoon chili paste

Spray a skillet with olive oil cooking spray. Over medium-high heat, stir-fry meat, chicken, or shrimp until cooked through. Remove to a plate. Turn off heat and spray pan with more olive oil spray. Over medium heat, stir-fry peppers, broccoli, celery, and sprouts. Cook until crisp-tender. Combine broth, soy sauce, and chili paste; stir into vegetables, add meat back into pan, and heat for 2–3 minutes. Makes 4 servings.

VEGGIE STIR-FRY

Olive oil cooking spray

1 red pepper, cut in 1-inch strips

1 yellow pepper, cut in 1-inch strips

1 green pepper, cut in 1-inch strips

1 cup broccoli florets, chopped

3 celery stalks, chopped

1 cup bean sprouts

½ cup fat-free, reduced-sodium chicken, beef, or vegetable broth

2 tablespoons low-sodium soy sauce

1 tablespoon chili paste

Optional: 1 cup (about 4 ounces) chopped cashews or peanuts (unsalted)

Spray a skillet with olive oil cooking spray. Over medium-high heat, stir-fry peppers, broccoli, celery, and sprouts. Cook until crisp-tender. Combine broth, soy sauce, and chili paste; stir into vegetables and heat for 1–2 minutes. Top with nuts (if using) and serve. Makes 4 servings.

GRILLED PORTOBELLO MUSHROOMS

2 large portobello mushrooms

Olive oil cooking spray

½ cup balsamic vinegar

½ teaspoon garlic, minced

2 tablespoons onion, chopped

2 tablespoons fresh basil, chopped

Clean the mushrooms and remove stems. Spray mushrooms lightly with olive oil cooking spray. In a small bowl, combine the balsamic vinegar, garlic, and onions. Marinate the mushrooms in this mixture for at least 1 hour. Pour mushrooms and marinade into a ceramic dish. Bake for 20–30 minutes, or until cooked through. Top mushrooms with fresh basil before serving. Makes 1 serving.

RATATOUILLE

Olive oil cooking spray

1 medium onion, chopped

2 garlic cloves, minced

1 eggplant, peeled and chopped

2 zucchinis, chopped

1 green pepper, chopped

1 medium tomato, chopped

¼ cup tomato juice

Parmesan cheese

Spray a large skillet with olive oil cooking spray. Add onion and garlic, and sauté 2–4 minutes, or until tender. Add eggplant, zucchini, green pepper, tomato, and tomato juice. Bring the mixture to a boil, then reduce heat to low. Simmer, covered, until vegetables are soft, stirring occasionally, about 8–10 minutes. Sprinkle with Parmesan cheese before serving. Makes 4 servings.

QUICK-FIX SPINACH LASAGNA

16 ounces low-fat cottage cheese

1 bag fresh spinach

1 egg

1 teaspoon crushed red pepper

Black pepper to taste

Olive oil cooking spray

8 ounces whole-wheat lasagna noodles, uncooked

1 cup marinara sauce

½ cup shredded mozzarella cheese

Preheat oven to 350 degrees. In a bowl, mix cottage cheese, spinach, egg, and red and black pepper. Spritz a baking dish with cooking spray. Spread out half the lasagna noodles. Cover with the cheese/spinach filling; top with the remaining noodles. Pour marinara sauce over the noodles; sprinkle with mozzarella cheese. Bake for 45-50 minutes. Serves 4.

(Optional: To cut down on carbs, skip the bottom layer of noodles.)

MASHED MAPLE CARROTS

1 pound carrots, peeled and sliced into coins

1 tablespoon maple syrup

1 teaspoon pumpkin pie spice

Boil the carrots in a saucepan of water for 40–45 minutes or until soft. Drain and mash carrots with a potato masher. Add the maple syrup and pumpkin pie spice; mix well. Reheat, if necessary, just before serving. Makes 4 servings.

GARLIC-ROSEMARY MASHED CAULIFLOWER

1 head cauliflower, cut into small pieces

2 tablespoons plain Greek yogurt

2 garlic cloves, minced

1 teaspoon fresh or dried rosemary, finely chopped

¼ cup Parmesan cheese

Boil the cauliflower in a saucepan of water for 6–8 minutes, or until very soft. Drain well. Using a blender or potato masher, puree or mash the cauliflower, yogurt, garlic, rosemary, and Parmesan cheese until smooth. Reheat, if necessary, before serving. Makes 4 servings.

ROASTED EGGPLANT

1 eggplant, peeled and cut into chunks

Vegetable cooking spray

1 teaspoon garlic, minced

1 teaspoon dried Italian herbs

Preheat oven to 350 degrees. Place the eggplant in a baking dish that has been sprayed with vegetable cooking spray. Sprinkle eggplant with garlic and herbs, then spray lightly with vegetable cooking spray. Bake about 20–30 minutes, or until tender. Makes 4 servings.

ROSEMARY SPINACH

Vegetable cooking spray

2 bags fresh spinach, washed

2 teaspoons fresh rosemary, chopped, or 1 teaspoon dried rosemary

Sprinkle of Parmesan cheese

Spray a skillet lightly with vegetable cooking spray. Add spinach and rosemary. Cook on low-medium heat until spinach is wilted. Top with Parmesan cheese. Makes 4 servings.

Recipes contain 1 High-Density Vegetable per serving.

Flex-Time Foods are listed as optional ingredients.

Unless otherwise indicated, recipes fit all plans
(STAT, RESTORE, and MAINTAIN).

ROASTED BABY REDS
(optional for RESTORE and MAINTAIN)

1 pound baby red potatoes

Olive oil cooking spray

Black pepper

Dried basil, rosemary, parsley, cumin, thyme, or whatever other dried herbs and spices you like

Preheat oven to 375 degrees. Wash and scrub potatoes. Cut each potato into quarter wedges (leave skin on). Place the potatoes on a cookie sheet that has been sprayed with olive oil cooking spray. Sprinkle black pepper and herbs or spices over potatoes. Spritz the potatoes with olive oil cooking spray. Bake 40–45 minutes, or until potatoes are tender. Makes 4 servings.

MEDITERRANEAN LIMA BEANS

1 16-ounce bag frozen lima beans

Olive oil cooking spray

2 tablespoons fresh thyme, chopped

¼ teaspoon black pepper

Sprinkle of Parmesan cheese

Microwave beans according to package directions. Drain. Place beans in a bowl; spray liberally with olive oil spray. Add thyme, pepper, and cheese and toss. Makes 4 servings.

BAKED SWEET POTATO FRIES

Olive oil cooking spray

1 pound sweet potatoes, cut into strips ½-inch thick, unpeeled

1 tablespoon olive oil

Dash of spices of your choice: chili powder and cumin; nutmeg and cinnamon; five-spice powder (Chinese); garam masala (Indian); Cajun seasoning, etc.

Preheat oven to 450 degrees. Spray medium baking sheet with olive oil spray. In a bowl, coat sweet potato strips with olive oil. Sprinkle on spices of your choice and mix well. Spread sweet potatoes in a single layer on the pan. Bake for 15 minutes. Remove pan from oven and flip the fries with a metal spatula. Bake 10–15 minutes longer, or until fries are nicely browned. Makes 4 servings.

DIPS AND SPREADS

ROSEMARY-GARLIC OLIVE OIL BREAD DIP

4 tablespoons extra-virgin olive oil

1 garlic clove, smashed (or more to taste)

½ teaspoon fresh or dried rosemary leaves, chopped fine (or more to taste)

Combine all ingredients. Makes 4 servings.

WHITE BEAN SPREAD

1 16-ounce can white beans, drained

2 garlic cloves

1 tablespoon olive oil

1 tablespoon plus 1 teaspoon fresh minced herbs, separated (use parsley, rosemary, thyme, cilantro, basil, or any other fresh herbs)

1 teaspoon lemon juice

Combine all ingredients except the 1 teaspoon minced fresh herbs in a food processor. Process until creamy. Spoon into a bowl; sprinkle with remaining herbs. Serve with fresh veggies, whole-grain bread, or whole-grain crackers.

GUACAMOLE

2 medium avocados, ripe

1 teaspoon lime juice

¼ cup red onion, diced

1 tomato, seeded and chopped

1 tablespoon cilantro, chopped

1 garlic clove, minced

Optional: ¼ jalapeño pepper, seeds removed, minced

Cut avocados in half, removing pit and scooping flesh into a bowl. Mash with a potato masher or fork. Mix in lime juice, onion, jalapeño (if using), tomato, cilantro, and garlic. Stir well. Makes 6 servings.

½ cup garbanzo beans, drained

1 tablespoon olive oil

Mash beans with a fork, then puree the beans and olive oil in a blender to make the spread. Serve on whole-wheat pita bread wedges. Makes 1 serving.

BIBLIOGRAPHY

INTRODUCTION

"American Heart Association Recommendations for Physical Activity in Adults." American Heart Association (AHA), September 11, 2013. http://www.heart.org/HEARTORG/GettingHealthy/PhysicalActivity/StartWalking/American-Heart-Association-Guidelines_UCM_307976_Article.jsp.

"Body Mass Index." Centers for Disease Control and Prevention (CDC). http://www.cdc.gov/healthyweight/assessing/bmi/.

"Body Mass Index Table." Centers for Disease Control and Prevention (CDC). http://www.nhlbi.nih.gov/guidelines/obesity/bmi_tbl.pdf.

Flegal, K. M., B. K. Kit, H. Orpana, and B. L. Graubard. "Association of All-Cause Mortality with Overweight and Obesity Using Standard Body Mass Index Categories: A Systematic Review and Meta-Analysis." *JAMA: Journal of the American Medical Association* 309, no. 1 (January 2, 2013): 71–82. http://jama.jamanetwork.com/article.aspx?articleid=1555137.

"How Much Physical Activity Do Adults Need?" Centers for Disease Control and Prevention (CDC). http://www.cdc.gov/physicalactivity/everyone/guidelines/adults.html.

Kaiser, Chris. "AHA Lauds AMA Call on Obesity." *MedPage Today*, June 21, 2013. http://www.medpagetoday.com/Cardiology/MetabolicSyndrome/40024.

"Overweight and Obesity Statistics." National Institute of Diabetes and Digestive and Kidney Diseases (NIDDK) Weight-Control Information Network. http://www.win.niddk.nih.gov/statistics/.

Pollack, Andrew. "AMA Recognizes Obesity as a Disease," *New York Times*, June 18, 2013. http://www.nytimes.com/2013/06/19/business/ama-recognizes-obesity-as-a-disease.html.

PART ONE

Cahill, L. E., S.E. Chiuve, R. A. Mekary, M. K. Jensen, A. J. Flint, F. B. Hu, and E. B. Rimm. "Prospective Study of Breakfast Eating and Incident Coronary Heart

Disease in a Cohort of Male US Health Professionals." *Circulation* 128, no. 4 (July 23, 2013): 337–43.
http://circ.ahajournals.org/content/128/4/337.long.

Dow, C. A., S. B. Going, H. H. Chow, B. S. Patil, and C. A. Thomson. "The Effects of Daily Consumption of Grapefruit on Body Weight, Lipids, and Blood Pressure in Healthy, Overweight Adults." *Metabolism* 61, no. 7 (July 2012): 1026–35.
http://www.ncbi.nlm.nih.gov/pubmed/22304836.

Fujioka, K., F. Greenway, J. Sheard, and Y. Ying. "The Effects of Grapefruit On Weight and Insulin Resistance: Relationship to the Metabolic Syndrome." *Journal of Medicinal Food* 9, no. 1 (Spring 2006): 49–54.
http://www.ncbi.nlm.nih.gov/pubmed/16579728.

Garaulet M., P. Gómez-Abellán, J. J. Alburquerque-Béjar, Y. C. Lee, J. M. Ordovás, and F. A. Scheer. "Timing of Food Intake Predicts Weight Loss Effectiveness." *International Journal of Obesity* 37, no. 4 (April 2013): 604–11.
http://www.ncbi.nlm.nih.gov/pubmed/23357955.

Jakubowicz, D., M. Barnea, J. Wainstein, O. Froy. "High Caloric Intake at Breakfast vs. Dinner Differentially Influences Weight Loss of Overweight and Obese Women." *Obesity*, March 20, 2013.
http://www.ncbi.nlm.nih.gov/pubmed/23512957.

Leidy, H. J., L. C. Ortinau, S. M. Douglas, and H. A. Hoertel. "Beneficial Effects of a Higher-Protein Breakfast on the Appetitive, Hormonal, and Neural Signals Controlling Energy Intake Regulation in Overweight/Obese, 'Breakfast-Skipping,' Late-Adolescent Girls." *American Journal of Clinical Nutrition* 97, no. 4 (April 2013): 677–88. http://ajcn.nutrition.org/content/97/4/677.long.

"Number of Americans with Diabetes Projected to Double or Triple by 2050." Centers for Disease Control and Prevention (CDC), October 22, 2010.
http://www.cdc.gov/media/pressrel/2010/r101022.html.

Odegaard, A. O., D. R. Jacobs Jr., L. M. Steffen, L. Van Horn, D. S. Ludwig, and M. A. Pereira. "Breakfast Frequency and Development of Metabolic Risk." *Diabetes Care*, June 17, 2013.
http://www.ncbi.nlm.nih.gov/pubmed/23775814.

Silver, H. J., M. S. Dietrich, and K. D. Niswender. "Effects of Grapefruit, Grapefruit Juice and Water Preloads on Energy Balance, Weight Loss, Body Composition, and Cardiometabolic Risk in Free-Living Obese Adults." *Nutrition and Metabolism*

8, no. 1 (February 2, 2011): 8. http://www.ncbi.nlm.nih.gov/pubmed/?term=effects+of+grapefruit%2C+grapefruit+juice%2C+and+water+preloads.

Smit, L. A., A. Baylin, and H. Campos. "Conjugated Linoleic Acid in Adipose Tissue and Risk of Myocardial Infarction." *American Journal of Clinical Nutrition* 92, no. 1 (July 2010): 34–40.
http://ajcn.nutrition.org/content/92/1/34.long.

PART TWO

Food Prescription #1: Eat With Your Mind

"Decrease Portion Sizes." United States Department of Agriculture (USDA).
http://www.choosemyplate.gov/weight-management-calories/weight-management/better-choices/decrease-portions.html.

"Portion Size." MedlinePlus, US National Library of Medicine (NLM).
http://www.nlm.nih.gov/medlineplus/ency/patientinstructions/000337.htm.

Food Prescription #2: Put Protein to Work for You

"A Guide to Choosing Protein Wisely." American Diabetes Association (ADA).
http://www.diabetes.org/mfa-recipes/tips/2012-03/your-complete-guide-to.html.

Astrup, A. "The Satiating Power of Protein—A Key to Obesity Prevention?" *American Journal of Clinical Nutrition* 82, no. 1 (July 2005) 1–2.
http://ajcn.nutrition.org/content/82/1/1.full.

"Cancer Experts Issue '5-Steps' Warning on Grilling Safety." American Institute for Cancer Research (AICR), May 6, 2013.
http://www.aicr.org/press/press-releases/5-steps-warning-grilling-safety.html.

Duckett, S. K., J. P. Neel, J. P. Fontenot, and W. M. Clapham. "Effects of Winter Stocker Growth Rate and Finishing System On: III. Tissue Proximate, Fatty Acid, Vitamin, and Cholesterol Content." *Journal of Animal Science* 87, no. 9 (September 2009): 2961–70.
http://www.journalofanimalscience.org/content/87/9/2961.long.

Due, A., S. Toubro, A. R. Skov, and A. Astrup. "Effect of Normal-Fat Diets, either Medium or High in Protein, on Body Weight in Overweight Subjects: A Randomised 1-Year Trial." *International Journal of Obesity Related Metabolic Disorders* 28,

no. 10 (October 2004): 1283–90.
http://www.ncbi.nlm.nih.gov/pubmed/15303109.

"Grill Smart This Season." American Institute for Cancer Research (AICR).
http://preventcancer.aicr.org/site/News2?id=15485.

Halton, T. L., and F. B. Hu. "The Effects of High Protein Diets on Thermogenesis, Satiety and Weight Loss: A Critical Review." *Journal of the American College of Nutrition* 23, no. 5 (October 2004): 373–85.
http://www.ncbi.nlm.nih.gov/pubmed/15466943.

Leidy, H. J., L. C. Ortinau, S. M. Douglas, and H. A. Hoertel. "Beneficial Effects of a Higher-Protein Breakfast on the Appetitive, Hormonal, and Neural Signals Controlling Energy Intake Regulation in Overweight/Obese, 'Breakfast-Skipping,' Late-Adolescent Girls." *American Journal of Clinical Nutrition* 97, no. 4 (April 2013): 677–88.
http://ajcn.nutrition.org/content/97/4/677.long.

McAfee, A. J., E. M. McSorley, G. J. Cuskelly, A. M. Fearon, B. W. Moss, J. A. Beattie, J. M. Wallace, M. P. Bonham, and J. J. Strain. "Red Meat from Animals Offered a Grass Diet Increases Plasma and Platelet n-3 PUFA in Healthy Consumers." *British Journal of Nutrition* 105, no. 1 (January 2011): 80–9.
http://www.ncbi.nlm.nih.gov/
pubmed/?term=red+meat+from+animals+offered+a+grass+diet+increases.

Navas-Carretero, S., I. Abete, M. A. Zulet, and J. A. Martínez. "Chronologically Scheduled Snacking with High-Protein Products within the Habitual Diet in Type-2 Diabetes Patients Leads to a Fat Mass Loss: A Longitudinal Study." *Nutrition Journal* 10 (July 14, 2011): 74.
http://www.nutritionj.com/content/10/1/74.

"Nutrition for Everyone: Protein." Centers for Disease Control and Prevention (CDC).
http://www.cdc.gov/nutrition/everyone/basics/protein.html.

Pan, A., Q. Sun, A. M. Bernstein, M. B. Schulze, J. E. Manson, M. J. Stampfer, W. C. Willett, and F. B. Hu. "Red Meat Consumption and Mortality: Results from 2 Prospective Cohort Studies." *Archives of Internal Medicine* 172, no. 7 (April 9, 2012): 555–63.
http://www.ncbi.nlm.nih.gov/pubmed/22412075.

"Protein: Moving Closer to Center Stage." Harvard School of Public Health (HSPH).
http://www.hsph.harvard.edu/nutritionsource/protein-full-story/.

"Seafood Health Facts: Making Smart Choices." Seafoodhealthfacts.org, a joint project of the Oregon State University, Cornell University, the Universities of Delaware, Rhode Island, Florida and California, and the Community Seafood Initiative. http://seafoodhealthfacts.org/.

Smith, J. S., F. Ameri, and P. Gadgil. "Effect of Marinades on the Formation of Heterocyclic Amines in Grilled Beef Steaks." *Journal of Food Science* 73, no. 6 (August 2008): T100–5.
http://www.ncbi.nlm.nih.gov/pubmed/19241593.

Weigle, D. S., P. A. Breen, C. C. Matthys, H. S. Callahan, K. E. Meeuws, V. R. Burden, and J. Q. Purnell. "A High-Protein Diet Induces Sustained Reductions in Appetite, Ad Libitum Caloric Intake, and Body Weight Despite Compensatory Changes in Diurnal Plasma Leptin and Ghrelin Concentrations." *American Journal of Clinical Nutrition* 82, no. 1 (July 2005): 41–48.
http://ajcn.nutrition.org/content/82/1/41.full.

Food Prescription #3: Choose Super-Filling, Fat-Burning Carbohydrates

"A Daily Dose of Antioxidants." USDA Agricultural Research Service.
http://www.ars.usda.gov/is/ar/archive/mar08/fruit0308.htm?pf=1.

"Carbohydrates." American Diabetes Association (ADA).
http://www.diabetes.org/food-and-fitness/food/what-can-i-eat/carbohydrates.html.

"Carbohydrates: The Bottom Line." Harvard School of Public Health (HSPH).
http://www.hsph.harvard.edu/nutritionsource/carbohydrates/.

"Fitness and Nutrition: Carbohydrates." Office of Women's Health, US Department of Health and Human Services.
http://womenshealth.gov/fitness-nutrition/nutrition-basics/carbohydrates.cfm#healthyUnhealthy.

Larsen, T. M., et al. "Diets with High or Low Protein Content and Glycemic Index for Weight-Loss Maintenance." *New England Journal of Medicine* 363, no. 22 (November 25 2010): 2102–13.
http://www.nejm.org/doi/pdf/10.1056/NEJMoa1007137.

Lennerz, B. S., D. C. Alsop, L. M. Holsen, E. Stern, R. Rojas, C. B. Ebbeling, J. M. Goldstein, and D. S. Ludwig. "Effects of Dietary Glycemic Index on Brain Regions Related to Reward and Craving in Men." *American Journal of Clinical Nutrition* 98, no. 3 (September 2013): 641–7. http://www.ncbi.nlm.nih.gov/pubmed/?term=effects+of+dietary+glycemic+index+on+brain+regions.

"Nutrition for Everyone: Carbohydrates." Centers for Disease Control and Prevention (CDC). http://www.cdc.gov/nutrition/everyone/basics/carbs.html.

Parker-Pope, Tara. "How Carbs Can Trigger Food Cravings." *New York Times*, June 27, 2013.
http://well.blogs.nytimes.com/2013/06/27/how-carbs-can-trigger-food-cravings/?ref=health&_r=1&pagewanted=print.

Food Prescription #4: Break Your Addiction to Sugar

Barclay, Eliza. "Sugar's Role in Rise of Diabetes Gets Clearer." *National Public Radio*, March 1, 2013.
http://www.npr.org/blogs/thesalt/2013/02/28/173170149/sugars-role-in-rise-of-diabetes-gets-clearer.

Hooper, L., A. Abdelhamid, H. J. Moore, W. Douthwaite, C. M. Skeaff, and C. D. Summerbell. "Effect of Reducing Total Fat Intake on Body Weight: Systematic Review and Meta-Analysis of Randomised Controlled Trials and Cohort Studies." *British Medical Journal* 345 (December 6, 2012): e7666.
http://www.ncbi.nlm.nih.gov/pubmed/23220130.

Lennerz, B. S., D. C. Alsop, L. M. Holsen, E. Stern, R. Rojas, C. B. Ebbeling, J. M. Goldstein, and D. S. Ludwig. "Effects of Dietary Glycemic Index on Brain Regions Related to Reward and Craving in Men." *American Journal of Clinical Nutrition* 98, no. 3 (September 2013): 641–7.
http://www.ncbi.nlm.nih.gov/pubmed/?term=effects+of+dietary+glycemic+index+on+brain+regions.

Lustig, Robert. "The Most Unhappy of Pleasures: This is Your Brain on Sugar." *Atlantic*, February 21, 2012.
http://www.theatlantic.com/health/archive/2012/02/the-most-unhappy-of-pleasures-this-is-your-brain-on-sugar/253341/.

Owens, Brian. "'Safe' Levels of Sugar Harmful to Mice." *Nature*, August 13, 2012.
http://www.nature.com/news/safe-levels-of-sugar-harmful-to-mice-1.13555.

Rada, P., N. M. Avena, and B. G. Hoebel. "Daily Bingeing on Sugar Repeatedly Releases Dopamine in the Accumbens Shell." *Neuroscience* 134, no. 3 (2005):737–44. http://www.ncbi.nlm.nih.gov/pubmed/15987666.

"Sugars and Carbohydrates." American Heart Association (AHA). http://www.heart.org/HEARTORG/GettingHealthy/NutritionCenter/Healthy-DietGoals/Sugars-and-Carbohydrates_UCM_303296_Article.jsp.

"Sugar and Desserts." American Diabetes Association (ADA). http://www.diabetes.org/food-and-fitness/food/what-can-i-eat/sweeteners-and-desserts.html.

"Sugary Drinks and Obesity Fact Sheet." Harvard School of Public Health (HSPH). http://www.hsph.harvard.edu/nutritionsource/sugary-drinks-fact-sheet/.

Swithers, S. E. "Artificial Sweeteners Produce the Counterintuitive Effect of Inducing Metabolic Derangements." *Trends in Endocrinology & Metabolism* 24, no. 9 (2013 July): 431–441. http://www.cell.com/trends/endocrinology-metabolism/fulltext/S1043-2760%2813%2900087-8.

Te Morenga, L., S. Mallard, and J. Mann. "Dietary Sugars and Body Weight: Systematic Review and Meta-Analyses of Randomised Controlled Trials and Cohort Studies." *British Medical Journal* 346 (January 15, 2012): e7492. http://www.ncbi.nlm.nih.gov/pubmed/?term=BMJ+2013%3B346%3Ae7492.

Food Prescription #5: Stop Fearing Fat

Astrup, A., J. Dyerberg, P. Elwood, K. Hermansen, F. B. Hu, M. U. Jakobsen, F. J. Kok, R. M. Krauss, J. M. Lecerf, P. LeGrand, P. Nestel, U. Risérus, T. Sanders, A. Sinclair, S. Stender, T. Tholstrup, and W. C. Willett. "The Role of Reducing Intakes of Saturated Fat in the Prevention of Cardiovascular Disease: Where Does the Evidence Stand in 2010?" *American Journal of Clinical Nutrition* 93, no. 4 (April 2011): 684–8. http://ajcn.nutrition.org/content/93/4/684.full.

"Avocado Nutrients." California Avocado Commission. http://www.californiaavocado.com/nutrition/.

"Eggs and Heart Disease." Harvard School of Public Health (HSPH).
http://www.hsph.harvard.edu/nutritionsource/eggs/.

"Fats and Cholesterol: Out with the Bad, In with the Good." HSPH.
http://www.hsph.harvard.edu/nutritionsource/fats-full-story/

Micha, R., and D. Mozaffarian. "Saturated Fat and Cardiometabolic Risk Factors, Coronary Heart Disease, Stroke, and Diabetes: A Fresh Look at the Evidence." *Lipids* 45 no. 10 (October 2010): 893–905.
http://www.ncbi.nlm.nih.gov/pmc/articles/PMC2950931/.

"Nutrition for Everyone: Dietary Cholesterol." Centers for Disease Control and Prevention (CDC).
http://www.cdc.gov/nutrition/everyone/basics/fat/cholesterol.html.

"Nutrition for Everyone: Dietary Fats." Centers for Disease Control and Prevention (CDC).
http://www.cdc.gov/nutrition/everyone/basics/fat/index.html.

"Nutrition for Everyone: Polyunsaturated Fats and Monounsaturated Fats." Centers for Disease Control and Prevention (CDC).
http://www.cdc.gov/nutrition/everyone/basics/fat/unsaturatedfat.html.

"Nutrition for Everyone: Saturated Fat." Centers for Disease Control and Prevention (CDC).
http://www.cdc.gov/nutrition/everyone/basics/fat/saturatedfat.html.

"Nutrition for Everyone: Trans Fat." Centers for Disease Control and Prevention (CDC).
http://www.cdc.gov/nutrition/everyone/basics/fat/transfat.html.

"Omega-3 Fatty Acids." University of Maryland Medical Center (UMMC).
http://umm.edu/health/medical/altmed/supplement/omega3-fatty-acids.

Siri-Tarino, P. W., Q. Sun, F. B. Hu, and R. M. Krauss. "Meta-Analysis of Prospective Cohort Studies Evaluating the Association of Saturated Fat with Cardiovascular Disease." *American Journal of Clinical Nutrition* 91, no. 3 (March 2010): 535–46.
http://ajcn.nutrition.org/content/91/3/535.full.

Food Prescription #6: Fill Your Plate with Vegetables and Food Prescription #7: Start Eating Fruit Again

Barone Gibbs, B., L. S. Kinzel, K. Pettee Gabriel, Y. F. Chang, and L. H. Kuller. "Short- and Long-Term Eating Habit Modification Predicts Weight Change in Overweight, Postmenopausal Women: Results from the WOMAN Study." *Journal of the Academy of Nutrition and Dietetics* 112, no. 9 (September 2012): 1347–1355, 1355.e1–2.
http://www.andjrnl.org/article/S2212-2672%2812%2900746-0/fulltext.

Bellavia, A., S. C. Larsson, M. Bottai, A. Wolk, and N. Orsini. "Fruit and Vegetable Consumption and All-Cause Mortality: A Dose-Response Analysis." *American Journal of Clinical Nutrition* 98, no. 2 (August 2013): 454–9.
http://ajcn.nutrition.org/content/early/2013/06/26/ajcn.112.056119.

"Can Eating Fruits and Vegetables Help People Manage Their Weight?" Centers for Disease Control and Prevention (CDC).
http://www.cdc.gov/nccdphp/dnpa/nutrition/pdf/rtp_practitioner_10_07.pdf.

"Carbohydrate Counting." American Diabetes Association (ADA).
http://www.diabetes.org/food-and-fitness/food/planning-meals/carb-counting/.

"Cruciferous Vegetables and Cancer Prevention." National Cancer Institute (NCI).
http://www.cancer.gov/cancertopics/factsheet/diet/cruciferous-vegetables.

Flood, J. E., and B. J. Rolls. "Soup Preloads in a Variety of Forms Reduce Meal Energy Intakes." *Appetite* 49, no. 3 (November 2007): 626–34.
http://www.ncbi.nlm.nih.gov/pubmed/17574705.

"Fruit or Vegetable: Do You Know the Difference?" Mayo Clinic, August 15, 2012.
http://www.mayoclinic.com/health/fruit-vegetable-difference/MY02201.

"Fruits." American Diabetes Association (ADA).
http://www.diabetes.org/food-and-fitness/food/what-can-i-eat/fruits.html.

"How to Use Fruits and Vegetables to Help Manage Your Weight." Centers for Disease Control and Prevention (CDC).
http://www.cdc.gov/healthyweight/healthy_eating/fruits_vegetables.html.

Kuehn, Bridget M. "Long-Term Weight Loss Aided by Boosting Fruit, Vegetable Consumption." *American Medical Association*, August 28, 2012.
http://newsatjama.jama.com/2012/08/28/
long-term-weight-loss-aided-by-boosting-fruit-vegetable-consumption/.

"Nutrition for Everyone: Fruits and Vegetables." Centers for Disease Control and Prevention (CDC).
http://www.cdc.gov/nutrition/everyone/fruitsvegetables/.

Parker-Pope, Tara. "Making the Case for Eating Fruit." *New York Times*, July 31, 2013.
http://well.blogs.nytimes.com/2013/07/31/making-the-case-for-eating-fruit/.

"State Indicator Report on Fruits and Vegetables, 2013." Centers for Disease Control and Prevention (CDC).
http://www.cdc.gov/nutrition/downloads/State-Indicator-Report-Fruits-Vegetables-2013.pdf.

"US Fruit and Vegetable Consumption: Who, What, Where, and How Much?" US Department of Agriculture (USDA).
http://www.ers.usda.gov/publications/aib-agricultural-information-bulletin/aib792-2.aspx#.UiDqx3_OBCo.

"What Foods Are in the Fruit Group?" US Department of Agriculture (USDA).
http://www.choosemyplate.gov/food-groups/fruits.html.

"What Foods Are in the Vegetable Group?" US Department of Agriculture (USDA).
http://www.choosemyplate.gov/food-groups/vegetables.html.

Whigham, L. D., A. R. Valentine, L. K. Johnson, Z. Zhang, R. L. Atkinson, and S. A. Tanumihardjo. "Increased Vegetable and Fruit Consumption during Weight Loss Effort Correlates with Increased Weight and Fat Loss." *Nutrition and Diabetes* 2 (October 1 2012): e48.
http://www.ncbi.nlm.nih.gov/pubmed/23449500.

"Why Is It Important to Eat Fruit?" US Department of Agriculture (USDA).
http://www.choosemyplate.gov/food-groups/fruits-why.html.

"Why Is It Important to Eat Vegetables?" US Department of Agriculture (USDA).
http://www.choosemyplate.gov/food-groups/vegetables-why.html.

Food Prescription #8: Go Nuts Over Nuts

Bes-Rastrollo, M., J. Sabaté, E. Gómez-Gracia, A. Alonso, J. A. Martínez, and M. A. Martínez-González. "Nut Consumption and Weight Gain in a Mediterranean Cohort: The SUN Study." *Obesity* 15, no. 1 (January 2007): 107–16. http://www.ncbi.nlm.nih.gov/pubmed/17228038.

Estruch, R., et al. "Primary Prevention of Cardiovascular Disease with a Mediterranean Diet." *New England Journal of Medicine* 368, no. 14 (April 4, 2013): 1279–90. http://www.ncbi.nlm.nih.gov/pubmed/23432189.

Guasch-Ferré, M., et al. "Frequency of Nut Consumption and Mortality Risk in the PREDIMED Nutrition Intervention Trial." *BMC Medicine* 11 (July 16, 2013): 164. http://www.ncbi.nlm.nih.gov/pubmed/23866098.

Jenkins, D. J., et al. "Nuts as a Replacement for Carbohydrates in the Diabetic Diet." *Diabetes Care* 34, no. 8 (August 2011): 1706–11. http://www.ncbi.nlm.nih.gov/pubmed/21715526.

Mattes, R. D., P. M. Kris-Etherton, and G. D. Foster. "Impact of Peanuts and Tree Nuts on Body Weight and Healthy Weight Loss in Adults." *Journal of Nutrition* 138, no. 9 (September 2008): 1741S–1745S. http://www.ncbi.nlm.nih.gov/pubmed/?term=impact+of+peanuts+and+tree+n+uts+on+body+weight.

Mozaffarian, D., T. Hao, E. B. Rimm, W. C. Willett, and F. B. Hu. "Changes in Diet and Lifestyle and Long-Term Weight Gain in Women and Men." *New England Journal of Medicine* 364, no. 25 (June 23, 2011): 2392–404. http://www.nejm.org/doi/full/10.1056/NEJMoa1014296.

"Nuts for the Heart." Harvard School of Public Health (HSPH). http://www.hsph.harvard.edu/nutritionsource/nuts-for-the-heart/.

Rohrmann, S., and D. Faeh. "Should We Go Nuts about Nuts?" *BMC Medicine* 11 (July 16, 2013): 165. http://www.ncbi.nlm.nih.gov/pubmed/23866107.

Sabaté, J., and Y. Ang. "Nuts and Health Outcomes: New Epidemiologic Evidence." *American Journal of Clinical Nutrition* 89, no. 5 (May 2009 May): 1643S–1648S. http://www.ncbi.nlm.nih.gov/pubmed/19321572.

Sabaté, J., K. Oda, and E. Ros. "Nut Consumption and Blood Lipid Levels: A Pooled Analysis of 25 Intervention Trials." *Archives of Internal Medicine* 170, no. 9 (May 10, 2010): 821–7.
http://www.ncbi.nlm.nih.gov/pubmed/20458092.

Food Prescription #9: Fall in Love with Legumes

Abete, I., D. Parra, and J. A. Martinez. "Legume-, Fish-, or High-Protein-Based Hypocaloric Diets: Effects on Weight Loss and Mitochondrial Oxidation in Obese Men." *Journal of Medicinal Food* 12, no. 1 (February 2009): 100–8.
http://www.ncbi.nlm.nih.gov//pubmed/19298202.

"Beans and Peas are Unique Foods." US Department of Agriculture (USDA).
http://www.choosemyplate.gov/food-groups/vegetables-beans-peas.html.

"Cooking Beans." US Dry Bean Council.
http://www.usdrybeans.com/recipes/cooking-beans/.

Curran, J. "The Nutritional Value and Health Benefits of Pulses in Relation to Obesity, Diabetes, Heart Disease and Cancer." *British Journal of Nutrition* 108, suppl. 1 (August 2012): S1–2.
http://www.ncbi.nlm.nih.gov/pubmed/22916804.

Jenkins, D. J., et al. "Effect of Legumes as Part of a Low Glycemic Index Diet on Glycemic Control and Cardiovascular Risk Factors in Type 2 Diabetes Mellitus: A Randomized Controlled Trial." *Archives of Internal Medicine* 172, no. 21 (November 26, 2012): 1653–60.
http://archinte.jamanetwork.com/article.aspx?articleid=1384247.

Nöthlings, U., et al. "Intake of Vegetables, Legumes, and Fruit, and Risk for All-Cause, Cardiovascular, and Cancer Mortality in a European Diabetic Population." *Journal of Nutrition* 138, no. 4 (April 2008): 775–81.
http://www.ncbi.nlm.nih.gov/pubmed/18356334.

Pan, A., Q. Sun, A. M. Bernstein, M. B. Schulze, J. E. Manson, M. J. Stampfer, W. C. Willett, and F. B. Hu. "Red Meat Consumption and Mortality: Results from 2 Prospective Cohort Studies." *Archives of Internal Medicine* 172, no. 7 (April 9, 2012): 555–63.
http://www.ncbi.nlm.nih.gov/pubmed/22412075.

Papanikolaou, Y., and V. L. Fulgoni III. "Bean Consumption Is Associated with

Greater Nutrient Intake, Reduced Systolic Blood Pressure, Lower Body Weight, and a Smaller Waist Circumference in Adults: Results from the National Health and Nutrition Examination Survey 1999–2002." *Journal of the American College of Nutrition* 27, no. 5 (October 2008): 569–76.
http://www.ncbi.nlm.nih.gov/pubmed/18845707.

Villegas, R., Y. T. Gao, G. Yang, H. L. Li, T. A. Elasy, W. Zheng, and X. O. Shu. "Legume and Soy Food Intake and the Incidence of Type 2 Diabetes in the Shanghai Women's Health Study." *American Journal of Clinical Nutrition* 87, no. 1 (January 2008): 162–7.
http://www.ncbi.nlm.nih.gov/pubmed/18175751.

Williams, P. G., S. J. Grafenauer, and J. E. O'Shea. "Cereal Grains, Legumes, and Weight Management: A Comprehensive Review of the Scientific Evidence." *Nutrition Reviews* 66, no. 4 (April 2008): 171–82.
http://www.ncbi.nlm.nih.gov/pubmed/18366531.

Zhang, Z., et al. "A High-Legume Low-Glycemic Index Diet Reduces Fasting Plasma Leptin in Middle-Aged Insulin-Resistant and -Sensitive Men." *European Journal of Clinical Nutrition* 65, no. 3 (March 2011): 415–8.
http://www.ncbi.nlm.nih.gov/pubmed/21206508.

Food Prescription #10: Go for Yogurt

"Changes in Specific Dietary Factors May Have Big Impact on Long-Term Weight Gain." Harvard School of Public Health (HSPH), June 22, 2011.
http://www.hsph.harvard.edu/news/press-releases/diet-lifestyle-weight-gain/.

Ejtahed, H. S., et al. "Effect of Probiotic Yogurt Containing Lactobacillus Acidophilus and Bifidobacterium Lactis on Lipid Profile in Individuals with Type 2 Diabetes Mellitus." *Journal of Dairy Science* 94, no. 7 (July 2011): 3288–94.
http://www.ncbi.nlm.nih.gov/pubmed/21700013.

Haupt, A., and K. Hiatt. "Greek Yogurt vs. Regular Yogurt: Which is More Healthful?" *US News and World Report*, September 30, 2011.
http://health.usnews.com/health-news/diet-fitness/diet/articles/2011/09/30/greek-yogurt-vs-regular-yogurt-which-is-more-healthful.

"Live and Active Culture Yogurt." National Yogurt Association.
http://aboutyogurt.com/Live-Culture.

Mozaffarian, D., T. Hao, E. B. Rimm, W. C. Willett, and F. B. Hu. "Changes in Diet and Lifestyle and Long-Term Weight Gain in Women and Men." *New England Journal of Medicine* 364, no. 25 (June 23, 2011): 2392–404. http://www.nejm.org/doi/full/10.1056/NEJMoa1014296.

"Promising Research Presented on Yogurt's Effects on Weight Management and Chronic Disease." American Society for Nutrition, June 18, 2013. http://asn-cdn-remembers.s3.amazonaws.com/4171dfcfb0a2ab4631f594e60e4e4778.pdf.

Smit, L. A., A. Baylin, and H. Campos. "Conjugated Linoleic Acid in Adipose Tissue and Risk of Myocardial Infarction." *American Journal of Clinical Nutrition* 92, no. 1 (July 2010): 34–40. http://ajcn.nutrition.org/content/92/1/34.long.

Stein, Rob. "Potatoes Bad, Nuts Good for Staying Slim, Harvard Study Finds." *Washington Post*, June 22, 2011. http://www.washingtonpost.com/national/health-science/potatoes-bad-nuts-good-for-staying-slim-harvard-study-finds/2011/06/17/AGRWmIgH_story.html.

Wang, H., K. A. Livingston, C. S. Fox, J. B. Meigs, and P. F. Jacques. "Yogurt Consumption Is Associated with Better Diet Quality and Metabolic Profile in American Men and Women." *Nutrition Research* 33, no. 1 (January 2013): 18–26. http://www.ncbi.nlm.nih.gov/pubmed/23351406.

Wang H., L. M. Troy, G. T. Rogers, C. S. Fox, N. M. McKeown, J. B. Meigs, and P. F. Jacques. "Longitudinal Association between Dairy Consumption and Changes of Body Weight and Waist Circumference: The Framingham Heart Study." *International Journal of Obesity*, May 20, 2013. http://www.ncbi.nlm.nih.gov/pubmed/23736371.

"Yogurt: Wholesome Food for Every Body." National Yogurt Association. http://aboutyogurt.com/index.asp?bid=31.

PART THREE

Weight-Loss Payoff #1: A Better YOU

"Causes and Consequences: What Causes Overweight and Obesity?" Centers for Disease Control and Prevention (CDC). http://www.cdc.gov/obesity/adult/causes/index.html.

Crowson, C. S., E. L. Matteson, J. M. Davis III, and S. E. Gabriel. "Contribution of Obesity to the Rise in Incidence of Rheumatoid Arthritis." *Arthritis Care & Research* 65, no. 1 (January 2013): 71–1.
http://www.ncbi.nlm.nih.gov/pubmed/22514156.

Hayashi, Annie. "Pearls and Pitfalls: Orthopaedics and Obesity." *AAOS Now*, June 2009.
http://www.aaos.org/news/aaosnow/jun09/clinical1.asp.

"Health Benefits of Losing Weight." National Library of Medicine PubMed Health.
http://www.ncbi.nlm.nih.gov/pubmedhealth/PMH0004993/.

Kane, Andrea. "How Fat Affects Arthritis." Arthritis Foundation.
http://www.arthritistoday.org/about-arthritis/arthritis-and-your-health/obesity/fat-and-arthritis.php.

Lawson, R., and B. Pruitt. "Issues in Obesity, Part 2: Obesity Weighs Heavily on Lung Function." *Nursing* 41, no. 11 (November 2011): 42–8.
http://www.nursingcenter.com/lnc/CEArticle?an=00152193-201111000-00014&Journal_ID=54016&Issue_ID=1246893.

Pollack, Peter. "Is There a Systemic Link Between Obesity and OA?" *AAOS Now*, March 2013.
http://www.aaos.org/news/aaosnow/mar13/clinical10.asp.

"Obesity Trends in Adults with Arthritis." Centers for Disease Control and Prevention (CDC).
http://www.cdc.gov/arthritis/resources/spotlights/obesity-trends.htm.

"Spotlight Obesity Trends: Obesity Trends in Adults with Arthritis." Centers for Disease Control and Prevention (CDC).
http://www.cdc.gov/arthritis/resources/spotlights/obesity-trends.htm.

"The Search for Alzheimer's Disease Causes and Risk Factors." Alzheimer's Association.
http://www.alz.org/research/science/alzheimers_disease_causes.asp.

"Weight Problems Take a Hefty Toll on Body and Mind." Harvard School of Public Health (HSPH).
http://www.hsph.harvard.edu/obesity-prevention-source/obesity-consequences/health-effects/.

"Causes of Diabetes." National Diabetes Information Clearinghouse (NDIC). http://diabetes.niddk.nih.gov/dm/pubs/causes/.

Colberg, S. R., et al. "Exercise and Type 2 Diabetes: The American College of Sports Medicine and the American Diabetes Association: Joint Position Statement." *Diabetes Care* 33, no. 12 (December 2010): e147–67. http://care.diabetesjournals.org/content/33/12/e147.abstract.

Colberg, S. R., L. Zarrabi, L. Bennington, A. Nakave, C. Thomas Somma, D. P. Swain, and S. R. Sechrist. "Postprandial Walking Is Better for Lowering the Glycemic Effect of Dinner Than Pre-Dinner Exercise in Type 2 Diabetic Individuals." *Journal of the American Medical Directors Association* 10, no. 6 (July 2009): 394–7. http://www.ncbi.nlm.nih.gov/pubmed/19560716.

"Diabetes Prevention Program (DPP)." National Diabetes Information Clearinghouse (NDIC). http://diabetes.niddk.nih.gov/dm/pubs/preventionprogram/index.aspx.

"Diabetes Statistics." American Diabetes Association (ADA). http://www.diabetes.org/diabetes-basics/diabetes-statistics/.

Dipietro, L., A. Gribok, M. S. Stevens, L. F. Hamm, and W. Rumpler. "Three 15-Min Bouts of Moderate Postmeal Walking Significantly Improves 24-H Glycemic Control in Older People at Risk for Impaired Glucose Tolerance." *Diabetes Care*, June 11, 2013. http://care.diabetesjournals.org/content/early/2013/06/03/dc13-0084.abstract.

Hu, F. B., J. E. Manson, M. J. Stampfer, et al. "Diet, Lifestyle, and the Risk of Type 2 Diabetes Mellitus in Women." *New England Journal of Medicine* 345 (2001):790–7. http://www.nejm.org/doi/full/10.1056/NEJMoa010492.

"Insulin Resistance and Pre-Diabetes." National Diabetes Information Clearinghouse (NDIC). http://diabetes.niddk.nih.gov/dm/pubs/insulinresistance/index.aspx.

"Simple Steps to Preventing Diabetes." Harvard School of Public Health (HSPH). http://www.hsph.harvard.edu/nutritionsource/preventing-diabetes-full-story/.

"The Facts About Diabetes: A Leading Cause of Death in the US." National Diabetes Education Program. http://ndep.nih.gov/diabetes-facts/index.aspx.

Weight-Loss Payoff #3: A Heart That Loves You

"American Heart Association Heart and Stroke Encyclopedia." American Heart Association (AHA).
http://www.heart.org/HEARTORG/Encyclopedia/Heart-Encyclopedia_UCM_445084_Encyclopedia.jsp?levelSelected=1.

Bankhead, Charles. "Fatal CHD Risk Soars with Obesity." *Medpage Today*, February 16, 2011.
http://www.medpagetoday.com/PrimaryCare/Obesity/24890.

"Coronary Artery Disease." Centers for Disease Control and Prevention (CDC).
http://www.cdc.gov/heartdisease/coronary_ad.htm.

Flegal, K. M., B. K. Kit, H. Orpana, and B. I. Graubard. "Association of All-Cause Mortality with Overweight and Obesity Using Standard Body Mass Index Categories: A Systematic Review and Meta-Analysis." *Journal of the American Medical Association* 309, no. 1 (2013): 71–82.
http://jama.jamanetwork.com/article.aspx?articleid=1555137.

Go, A. S., et al. "Heart Disease and Stroke Statistics—2013 Update. A Report from the American Heart Association." *Circulation* 127 (2013): e6-e245.
http://circ.ahajournals.org/content/127/1/e6.full.pdf+html.

"Heart Attack." Centers for Disease Control and Prevention (CDC).
http://www.cdc.gov/heartdisease/heart_attack.htm.

"Heart Disease." Mayo Clinic.
http://www.mayoclinic.com/health/heart-disease/DS0112.

"Heart Disease Facts." Centers for Disease Control and Prevention (CDC).
http://www.cdc.gov/heartdisease/facts.htm.

"Heart Disease Prevention: What You Can Do. Live a Healthy Lifestyle." Centers for Disease Control and Prevention (CDC).
http://www.cdc.gov/heartdisease/what_you_can_do.htm.

"How Can I Lower High Cholesterol?" American Heart Association (AHA).
http://www.heart.org/idc/groups/heart-public/@wcm/@hcm/documents/downloadable/ucm_300460.pdf.

Kenchaiah, S., J. C. Evans, D. Levy, et al. "Obesity and the Risk of Heart Failure."

New England Journal of Medicine 347, no. 5 (August 1, 2002): 305–313.
http://www.nejm.org/doi/full/10.1056/NEJMoa020245.

Logue, J., H. M. Murray, P. Welsh, J. Shepherd, C. Packard, P. Macfarlane, S. Cobbe, I. Ford, and N. Sattar. "Obesity Is Associated with Fatal Coronary Heart Disease Independently of Traditional Risk Factors and Deprivation." *Heart* 97 (2011): 564–568.
http://heart.bmj.com/content/97/7/564.short.

Nicklas, B. J., M. Cesari, B. W. Penninx, et al. "Abdominal Obesity Is an Independent Risk Factor for Chronic Heart Failure in Older People. *Journal of the American Geriatric Society* 54, no. 3 (2006): 413–420.
http://www.ncbi.nlm.nih.gov/pubmed/16551307.

"Numbers that Count for a Healthy Heart." American Heart Association (AHA).
http://www.heart.org/idc/groups/heart-public/@wcm/@hcm/documents/download-able/ucm_428691.pdf.

"Obesity Information from the American Heart Association." American Heart Association (AHA).
http://www.heart.org/HEARTORG/GettingHealthy/WeightManagement/Obesi-ty/Obesity-Information_UCM_307908_Article.jsp.

Stevens, V. J., et al. "Long-Term Weight Loss and Changes in Blood Pressure: Results of the Trials of Hypertension Prevention, Phase II." *Annals of Internal Medicine* 134, no. 1 (2001): 1–11.
http://annals.org/article.aspx?articleid=714088.

"Waist Size Matters." Harvard School of Public Health (HSPH).
http://www.hsph.harvard.edu/obesity-prevention-source/obesity-definition/abdominal-obesity/.

"What Are the Health Risks of Overweight and Obesity?" National Heart, Lung, and Blood Institute (NHLBI).
http://www.nhlbi.nih.gov/health/health-topics/topics/obe/risks.html.

"What Is High Blood Pressure?" American Heart Association (AHA).
http://www.heart.org/HEARTORG/Conditions/HighBloodPressure/AboutHigh-BloodPressure/What-is-High-Blood-Pressure_UCM_301759_Article.jsp.

Weight-Loss Payoff #4: A Major Cool-Down of Chronic Inflammation

Bauer, Brent. "Buzzed on Inflammation." *Mayo Clinic Health Letter Online Edition*, 2013.
http://healthletter.mayoclinic.com/editorial/editorial.cfm/i/163/t/Buzzed%20
on%20inflammation/.

Flaherty, Julie. "Lose Weight and Boost Immunity." *Tufts Journal*, May 26, 2010.
http://tuftsjournal.tufts.edu/2010/05_2/features/04/.

Galland, L. "Diet and inflammation." *Nutrition Clinical Practice* 25, no. 6 (December 2010): 634–40.
http://www.ncbi.nlm.nih.gov/pubmed/21139128.

Giugliano, D., A. Ceriello, and K. Esposito. "The Effects of Diet on Inflammation: Emphasis on the Metabolic Syndrome." *Journal of the American College of Cardiologists* 48, no. 4 (2006): 677–685.
http://content.onlinejacc.org/article.aspx?articleid=1137818.

Imayama, I., C. M. Ulrich, C. M. Alfano, C. Wang, L. Xiao, M. H. Wener, K. L. Campbell, C. Duggan, K. E. Foster-Schubert, A. Kong, C. E. Mason, C. Y. Wang, G. L. Blackburn, C. E. Bain, H. J. Thompson, and A. McTiernan. "Effects of a Caloric Restriction Weight Loss Diet and Exercise on Inflammatory Biomarkers in Overweight/Obese Postmenopausal Women: A Randomized Controlled Trial." *Cancer Research* 72, no. 9 (May 1, 2012): 2314–26.
http://cancerres.aacrjournals.org/content/72/9/2314.long.

"Inflammation and Heart Disease." American Heart Association (AHA).
http://www.heart.org/HEARTORG/Conditions/Inflammation-and-Heart-Disease_UCM_432150_Article.jsp.

Jenson, P., et al. "Effect of Weight Loss on the Severity of Psoriasis: A Randomized Clinical Study." *JAMA Dermatology* 149, no. 7 (2013): 795–801.
http://archderm.jamanetwork.com/article.aspx?articleid=1690928.

Johnson, A. R., J. J. Milner, and L. Makowski. "The Inflammation Highway: Metabolism Accelerates Inflammatory Traffic in Obesity." *Immunological Reviews* 249, no. 1 (September 2012): 218–38.
http://www.ncbi.nlm.nih.gov/pubmed/22889225.

Karlsson, E. A., and M. A. Beck. "The Burden of Obesity on Infectious Disease." *Experimental Biology Medicine* 235, no. 12 (December 2010): 1412–24.

http://www.ncbi.nlm.nih.gov/pubmed/21127339.

Kotz, Deborah. "Building a Diet that Lowers Inflammation." *US News and World Report*, November 2, 2009.
http://health.usnews.com/health-news/diet-fitness/articles/2009/11/02/building-a-diet-that-lowers-inflammation_print.html.

Landro, Laura. "The New Science Behind America's Deadliest Diseases." *Wall Street Journal*, July 16, 2012.
http://online.wsj.com/article/SB100014240527023036128045775310924535900 70.html.

Milner, J. J., and M. A. Beck. "The Impact of Obesity on the Immune Response to Infection." *Proceedings of the Nutrition Society* 71, no. 2 (May 2012): 298–306.
http://www.ncbi.nlm.nih.gov/pubmed/22414338.

Sheridan, P. A., et al. "Obesity is Associated with Impaired Immune Response to Influenza Vaccination in Humans." *International Journal of Obesity* 36 (October 25, 2012: 1072–1077.
http://www.nature.com/ijo/journal/v36/n8/full/ijo2011208a.html.

Van Wayenburg C. A. M., et al. "Encounters for Common Illnesses in General Practice Increased in Obese Patients." *Family Practice* 25, suppl. 1 (December 2008): i93-8.
http://fampra.oxfordjournals.org/content/25/suppl_1/i93.long.

"What Is Inflammation? What Causes Inflammation?" *Medical News Today*, July 31, 2012. http://www.medicalnewstoday.com/articles/248423.php.

"What You Eat Can Fuel or Cool Inflammation, A Key Driver of Heart Disease, Diabetes, and Other Conditions." *Harvard Medical School Family Health Guide*.
http://www.health.harvard.edu/fhg/updates/What-you-eat-can-fuel-or-cool-inflammation-a-key-driver-of-heart-disease-diabetes-and-other-chronic-conditions.shtml.

Weight-Loss Payoff #5: More Satisfying Sleep

Anglin, R. E., Z. Samaan, S. D. Walter, and S. D. McDonald. "Vitamin D Deficiency and Depression in Adults: Systematic Review and Meta-Analysis." *British Journal of Psychiatry* 202 (February 2013: 100–7.
http://www.ncbi.nlm.nih.gov/pubmed/23377209.

Blumenthal, J. A., P. J. Smith, and B. M. Hoffman. "Is Exercise a Viable Treatment for Depression?" *ACSM's Health and Fitness Journal* 16, no. 4 (July 2012): 14–21. http://www.ncbi.nlm.nih.gov/pubmed/23750100.

Fabricatore, A. N., T. A. Wadden, A. J. Higginbotham, L. F. Faulconbridge, A. M. Nguyen, S. B. Heymsfield, M. S. Faith. "Intentional Weight Loss and Changes in Symptoms of Depression: A Systematic Review and Meta-Analysis." *International Journal of Obesity* 35, no. 11 (November 2011): 1363–76. http://www.ncbi.nlm.nih.gov/pubmed/21343903.

Faulconbridge, L. F., T. A. Wadden, et al. "One-Year Changes in Symptoms of Depression and Weight in Overweight/Obese Individuals with Type 2 Diabetes in the Look AHEAD Study." *Obesity* 20, no. 4 (April 2012): 783–93. http://www.ncbi.nlm.nih.gov/pubmed/22016099.

"Magnesium." NIH Office of Dietary Supplements Dietary Supplement Fact Sheet. http://dietary-supplements.info.nih.gov/factsheets/magnesium.asp.

Nielsen, Forrest. "Do You Ever Have Trouble Sleeping? More Magnesium Might Help." *USDA Agricultural Research Service News,* July 9, 2007. http://www.ars.usda.gov/News/docs.htm?docid=15617.

Pase, M. P., A. B. Scholey, A. Pipingas, M. Kras, K. Nolidin, A. Gibbs, K. Wesnes, and C. Stough. "Cocoa Polyphenols Enhance Positive Mood States but Not Cognitive Performance: A Randomized, Placebo-Controlled Trial." *Journal of Psychopharmacology* 27, no. 5 (May 2013): 451–8. http://jop.sagepub.com/content/27/5/451.long.

Pittman, Genevra. "Weight Loss Programs May Boost Mood in Obese People." *Reuters Health,* March 7, 2011. http://www.reuters.com/article/2011/03/07/us-weight-loss-people-idUSTRE7264TV20110307.

Platte, P., C. Herbert, P. Pauli, and P. A. Breslin. "Oral Perceptions of Fat and Taste Stimuli Are Modulated by Affect and Mood Induction." *PLoS One* 8, no. 6 (June 5, 2013): e65006. http://www.ncbi.nlm.nih.gov/pubmed/23755167.

"Selenium." NIH Office of Dietary Supplements Dietary Supplement Fact Sheet. http://dietary-supplements.info.nih.gov/factsheets/selenium.asp.

"Selenium Can Lift the Spirits." USDA Agricultural Research Service.
http://www.ars.usda.gov/News/docs.htm?docid=15617.

Swayne, Matthew. "Unhealthy Eating Can Make a Bad Mood Worse." *Penn State News*, March 15, 2013.
http://news.psu.edu/story/268780/2013/03/15/research/
unhealthy-eating-can-make-bad-mood-worse.

"Tryptophan." National Library of Medicine Medical Encyclopedia.
http://www.nlm.nih.gov/medlineplus/ency/article/002332.htm.

"Vitamin D." NIH Office of Dietary Supplements Dietary Supplement Fact Sheet.
http://ods.od.nih.gov/factsheets/VitaminD-HealthProfessional/.

Weir, K. "The Exercise Effect." *Monitor on Psychology* 42, no. 11 (December 2011): 48. http://www.apa.org/monitor/2011/12/exercise.aspx.

Weight-Loss Payoff #6: Higher Energy and a Happier Mood

"Body Weight and Cancer Risk." American Cancer Society (ACS).
http://www.cancer.org/acs/groups/cid/documents/webcontent/002578-pdf.pdf.

"Body Weight and Weight Gain." Susan G. Komen for the Cure.
http://ww5.komen.org/breastcancer/overweightweightgain.html.

"Cancer Facts and Figures 2013." American Cancer Society (ACS).
http://www.cancer.org/acs/groups/content/@epidemiologysurveilance/documents/
document/acspc-036845.pdf.

"Cancer Trends Progress Report—2011/2012 Update." National Cancer Institute.
http://progressreport.cancer.gov/doc_detail.
asp?pid=1&did=2007&chid=71&coid=709&mid=.

"Food, Nutrition, Physical Activity, and the Prevention of Cancer: A Global Perspective." World Cancer Research Fund and the American Institute for Cancer Research.
http://eprints.ucl.ac.uk/4841/1/4841.pdf.

"From Prevention to Survivorship: The Obesity-Cancer Challenge."
MD Anderson Cancer Center. http://www.newswise.com/articles/
from-prevention-to-survivorship-the-obesity-cancer-challenge.

"Harms of Smoking and Health Benefits of Quitting." National Cancer Institute (NCI). http://www.cancer.gov/cancertopics/factsheet/Tobacco/cessation.

Imayama, I., C. M. Ulrich, C. M. Alfano, C. Wang, L. Xiao , M. H. Wener, K. L. Campbell, C. Duggan, K. E. Foster-Schubert, A. Kong, C. E. Mason, C. Y. Wang, G. L. Blackburn, C. E. Bain, H. J. Thompson, and A. McTiernan. "Effects of a Caloric Restriction Weight Loss Diet and Exercise on Inflammatory Biomarkers in Overweight/Obese Postmenopausal Women: A Randomized Controlled Trial." *Cancer Research* 72, no. 9 (May 1, 2012): 2314–26.
http://cancerres.aacrjournals.org/content/72/9/2314.long.

"Link Between Obesity and Cancer." Proceedings of the National Academy of Sciences.
http://www.pnas.org/content/110/22/8753.full.

"Obesity and Cancer Risk." National Cancer Institute (NCI).
http://www.cancer.gov/cancertopics/factsheet/Risk/obesity.

"Physical Activity and Cancer." National Cancer Institute (NCI).
http://www.cancer.gov/cancertopics/factsheet/prevention/physicalactivity.

Teras, L. R., M. Goodman, A. V. Patel, W. R. Diver, W. D. Flanders, and H. S. Feigelson. "Weight Loss and Postmenopausal Breast Cancer in a Prospective Cohort of Overweight and Obese US Women." *Cancer Causes and Control* 22, no. 4 (April 2011): 573–9.
http://www.ncbi.nlm.nih.gov/pubmed/21327461.

"The Obesity-Cancer Connection, and What We Can Do About It." American Cancer Society (ACS).
http://www.cancer.org/cancer/news/expertvoices/post/2013/02/28/the-obesity-cancer-connection-and-what-we-can-do-about-it.aspx.

Vucenik, I., and J. P. Stains. "Obesity and Cancer Risk: Evidence, Mechanisms, and Recommendations." *Annals of the New York Academy of Sciences* 1271 (October 2012): 37–43.
http://onlinelibrary.wiley.com/doi/10.1111/j.1749-6632.2012.06750.x/pdf.

Weight-Loss Payoff #7: A Lower Risk of Cancer

Mitchell, J. A., D. Rodriguez, K. H. Schmitz, J. Audrain-McGovern. "Sleep Duration and Adolescent Obesity." *Pediatrics* 131, no. 5 (May 2013): e1428–34.

http://www.ncbi.nlm.nih.gov/pubmed/23569090.

"Night Owls May Pack on More Pounds." *MedLine Plus HealthDay*, June 28, 2013. http://www.nlm.nih.gov/medlineplus/news/fullstory_138271.html.

"Obesity and Sleep." National Sleep Foundation. http://www.sleepfoundation.org/article/sleep-topics/obesity-and-sleep.

Parker-Pope, Tara. "Cheating Ourselves of Sleep." *New York Times*, June 17, 2013. http://well.blogs.nytimes.com/2013/06/17/cheating-ourselves-of-sleep/?pagewanted=print.

Parker-Pope, Tara. "How Sleep Loss Adds to Weight Gain." *New York Times*, August 6, 2013. http://well.blogs.nytimes.com/2013/08/06/how-sleep-loss-adds-to-weight-gain/?smid=tw-nytimeshealth&seid=auto&_r=0.

Patel, S. R., A. Malhotra, D. P. White, D. J. Gottlieb, and F. B. Hu. "Association between Reduced Sleep and Weight Gain in Women." *American Journal of Epidemiology* 164 (2006): 947–54. http://www.ncbi.nlm.nih.gov/pubmed/16914506.

Patel, S. R., F. B. Hu. "Short Sleep Duration and Weight Gain: A Systematic Review." *Obesity 16* (2008): 643–53. http://www.ncbi.nlm.nih.gov/pubmed/18239586.

"Sleep: Waking Up to Sleep's Role in Weight Control." Harvard School of Public Health (HSPH). http://www.hsph.harvard.edu/obesity-prevention-source/obesity-causes/sleep-and-obesity/.

"Sleep Disorders & Insufficient Sleep: Improving Health through Research." National Heart, Lung, and Blood Institute (NHLBI). http://www.nhlbi.nih.gov/news/spotlight/fact-sheet/sleep-disorders-insufficient-sleep-improving-health-through-research.html.

"What Is Sleep Apnea?" National Heart, Lung, and Blood Institute (NHLBI). http://www.nhlbi.nih.gov/health/health-topics/topics/sleepapnea/.

"Who Is at Risk for Sleep Apnea?" National Heart, Lung, and Blood Institute (NHLBI). http://www.nhlbi.nih.gov/health/health-topics/topics/sleepapnea/atrisk.html.

Yu, J. C., and P. Berger III. "Sleep Apnea and Obesity." *South Dakota Medicine*, spec. no. (2011): 28–34. http://www.ncbi.nlm.nih.gov/pubmed/21717814.

Weight-Loss Payoff #8: A Healthier Family Now—And for Generations to Come

"Alzheimer's Causes and Risk Factors." Alzheimer's Association. http://www.alz. org/espanol/about/causes_and_risk_factors.asp#other.

"Childhood Obesity Facts." Centers for Disease Control and Prevention (CDC). http://www.cdc.gov/healthyyouth/obesity/facts.htm.

Duffey, K. J., P. Gordon-Larsen, L. M. Steffen, D. R. Jacobs Jr., and B. M. Popkin. "Regular Consumption from Fast Food Establishments Relative to Other Restaurants Is Differentially Associated with Metabolic Outcomes in Young Adults." *Journal of Nutrition* 139, no. 11 (November 2009): 2113–8. http://www.ncbi.nlm.nih.gov/pubmed/19776183.

"Family, Friends Can Influence Weight and Mood." *Harvard Men's Health Watch*, December 2011. http://www.health.harvard.edu/press_releases/ family-friends-can-influence-weight-and-mood.

"Food and Diet." Harvard School of Public Health (HSPH). http://www.hsph.harvard.edu/obesity-prevention-source/obesity-causes/ diet-and-weight/#portion-size-and-weight-control.

Golan, R., D. Schwarzfuchs, M. J. Stampfer, I. Shai, and DIRECT group. "Halo Effect of a Weight-Loss Trial on Spouses: The DIRECT-Spouse Study." *Public Health Nutrition* 13, no. 4 (April 2010): 544–9. http://www.ncbi.nlm.nih.gov/pubmed/19706214.

Harder, T., E. Rodekamp, K. Schellong, J. W. Dudenhausen, and A. Plagemann. "Birth Weight and Subsequent Risk of Type 2 Diabetes: A Meta-Analysis." *American Journal of Epidemiology* 165, no. 8 (April 15, 2007): 849–57. http://www.ncbi.nlm.nih.gov/pubmed/17215379.

Huxley, R., C. G. Owen, P. H. Whincup, D. G. Cook, J. Rich-Edwards, G. D. Smith, and R. Collins. "Is Birth Weight a Risk Factor for Ischemic Heart Disease in Later Life?" *American Journal of Clinical Nutrition* 85, no. 5 (May 2007): 1244-50. http://www.ncbi.nlm.nih.gov/pubmed/17490959.

Landhuis, C. E., R. Poulton, D. Welch, and R. J. Hancox. "Childhood Sleep Time and Long-Term Risk for Obesity: A 32-Year Prospective Birth Cohort Study." *Pediatrics* 122, no. 5 (November 2008): 955–60. http://www.ncbi.nlm.nih.gov/pubmed/18977973.

"Limiting Pregnancy Weight Gain Could Benefit Infants' Health." American Diabetes Association (ADA). http://www.diabetes.org/news-research/research/access-diabetes-research/limiting-pregnancy-weight.html.

Ludwig, D. S., and J. Currie. "The Association between Pregnancy Weight Gain and Birthweight: A Within-Family Comparison." *Lancet* 376, no. 9745 (September 18, 2010): 984–990. http://www.ncbi.nlm.nih.gov/pubmed/20691469.

Meltzer, A. L., S. A. Novak, J. K. McNulty, E. A. Butler, and B. R. Karney. "Marital Satisfaction Predicts Weight Gain in Early Marriage." *Health Psychology* 32, no. 7 (July 2013): 824–7. http://www.ncbi.nlm.nih.gov/pubmed/23477578.

Mitchell, J. A., D. Rodriguez, K. H. Schmitz, and J. Audrain-McGovern. "Greater Screen Time Is Associated with Adolescent Obesity: A Longitudinal Study of the BMI Distribution from Ages 14 to 18." *Obesity* 21, no. 3 (March 2013): 572–5. http://www.ncbi.nlm.nih.gov/pubmed/23592665.

Reilly, J. J., et al. "Early Life Risk Factors for Obesity in Childhood: Cohort Study." *British Medical Journal* 330, no. 7504 (June 11, 2005): 1357. http://www.ncbi.nlm.nih.gov/pubmed/15908441.

"The Overweight Pet: How to Identify and Assist Your Overweight (or Obese) Dog." PetMD. http://www.petmd.com/dog/nutrition/evr_dg_identify_overweight_pet#.UiTI5H_OBCp.

"Weight Gain During Pregnancy." March of Dimes. http://www.marchofdimes.com/pregnancy/print/weight-gain-during-pregnancy.html.

Ziol-Guest, K. M., R. E. Dunifon, and A. Kalil. "Parental Employment and Children's Body Weight: Mothers, Others, and Mechanisms." *Social Science and Medicine*, September 14, 2012. http://www.ncbi.nlm.nih.gov/pubmed/23031605.